D0467163

Discover the Power of Meridian Tapping

A Revolutionary Method for Stress-Free Living

by Patricia Carrington, Ph.D.

Companion book to the movie *The Tapping Solution*
created and produced by Nicolas Ortner

The Tapping Solution
39 Beverly Dr.
Brookfield, CT 06804

Discover the Power of Meridian Tapping
A Revolutionary Method for Stress-Free Living
Copyright © 2008 by Patricia Carrington

Edited by Andrew Wolfendon

All rights reserved.
No part of this publication may be reproduced, stored
in a retrieval system, or transmitted in any form, by any
means, electronically, mechanically, photo copying,
recording or otherwise, without the prior written
permission of the publishers.

ISBN 978-0-615-41700-4

CONTENTS

The Reason This Book Was Written   v
Some Words of Thanks   xi

Part 1 The Story of Meridian Tapping

1 Too Good To Be True?   3
2 It's All About Energy   11
3 Science Faces a Revolution   19
4 Tapping's Family Tree   24
5 A Look at the Proof   29

Part 2 Learning Meridian Tapping

6 Basic Steps (the How To Chapter)   37
7 Uncovering Hidden Aspects While Tapping   52
8 It's Good to Have a Choice   58
9 Meridian Tapping for Past, Present and Future   67

Part 3 Using Meridian Tapping

10 Try Tapping for Fears and Phobias   77
11 Try Tapping to Enhance Performance   94
12 Try Tapping to Improve Weight Loss   113
13 Try Tapping for Physical Conditions and Pain   128
14 Try Tapping for Just About Everything   143

Part 4 The 4-Day Tapping Retreat

15 Overview   161
16 Bernadette's Story   164
17 Dennis's Story   169
18 Donna's Story   174
19 Jackie's Story   179
20 Jodi's Story   184
21 Jon's Story   190
22 Patricia's Story   196
23 Rene's Story   202
24 Sam's Story   207
25 Thea's Story   213

PART 5 What to Expect

26 The Future of Meridian Tapping   221

Special Resources   227
References   232

The Reason This Book was Written

New "self improvement" and alternative health methods are bursting on the scene almost weekly. Each of them holds out a bold promise for transforming some aspect of our lives — our physical health, our emotional well-being, our spiritual awareness, the quality of our relationships, or almost any other area of concern we might possibly have are addressed. We are bombarded by new hope-building possibilities.

Though most of us greet with enthusiasm any authentic new opportunity for self improvement and better health, we can also find ourselves overwhelmed by this and uncertain and confused by the barrage of offerings. We're like the over-stimulated shopper staring at a wall of endless options.

Which of these techniques should we be using? Is there a special one that will really tackle our unique personal problems? Will reading a particular book or doing a special exercise really change our lives? And when we run into conflicting information, such as often appears in the field of health and nutrition, whom and what should we believe? The average person can become discouraged.

As a result, many of us tend to dabble in one method for a brief time, see that we're not getting results right away, and then jump into another technique — and another one, and another, and so on. In the end we may throw up our hands and declare that, "nothing works," and that everything out there is being "sold" to us. Or we simply decide we don't have enough time to change our health or finances or relationships or whatever the issue may be. "If I only had ten free hours a week, then perhaps I could meditate or exercise more or call my mother more often…"

Those of us who do commit to a specific technique often worry whether we are using it correctly or implementing the concept in the "right" way. I hear the frustration in people's voices when they tell me, "I learned all about that stuff and gave it my best, but it doesn't seem to work!"

Anyone who is seriously engaged in helping others today, be they an author, a motivational speaker, a nutritionist, a counselor, or any type of trainer, teacher or leader, therefore faces a major credibility problem. The information overload is in danger of destroying our ability to help.

Nevertheless, I find that our world seems to work in a remarkable way — whenever we are confronted with new, more challenging problems, we seem to find new, more effective solutions.

For me, and for a great many of my friends and colleagues, meridian tapping is one of these solutions. It is a genuine breakthrough in the field of human development, one so surprising that those operating under our current paradigm often exclaim, "There's no way this can be for real!"

I sympathize with their skepticism. When you witness someone who has suffered knee pain for 15 years permanently erase it after forty-five minutes of tapping, part of your mind shouts, "That can't be true!" Or when you hear of someone with a lifelong snake phobia clearing it up within five minutes to an hour, it seems impossible. Our traditional understanding of such conditions is that they take years of therapeutic work and that their treatment is a slow and tortuous process.

What is amazing about meridian tapping — often referred to as simply "tapping" — is that we don't have to work to convince you or anyone else of its ability to change your life. If you're willing to try it for even a few minutes, you'll convince yourself! You can have a direct experience that shows you that it works! That's how simple tapping is and why it is spreading so rapidly throughout the world. One person after another tries it, experiences success, and then just "has to" tell a friend about it.

I personally came to learn about meridian tapping through that great source of information (and information overload!), the internet. It was there that I discovered the fascinating material that Gary Craig, the creator of an important tapping technique, Emotional Freedom Techniques, provides on his website and in his teaching materials. After reading and learning everything I could about EFT, I started applying it to my own life and sharing it with friends and family. I then experienced, first-hand, how quickly it worked to clear up, often permanently, a wide variety of issues in my life, from a simple crick in my neck to persistent procrastination on a new project, as well as many others.

The exciting thing was that EFT (as well as other forms of meridian tapping) was not one of those hyped up "New Age" products, infused with jargon and ritual, high on promise, low on real-world results. The strength of the meridian tapping material, including the rapidly accumulating literature on EFT, is its wealth of real-life reports from people who have successfully used tapping on a wide variety of fears, pains, mental/emotional obstacles and other serious life issues. Meridian tapping is not a fad but a genuinely effective and revolutionary way of changing human emotions and behaviors for the better.

My personal experience with tapping turned out to be so impressive, in fact, that I soon felt a strong need to document this approach in some manner so that others could experience its impact as I had. Simply telling people wasn't enough. I wanted to show them what tapping can actually do.

The solution I came up with was to make a documentary film. Although I had no knowledge of filmmaking and zero financial backing for a project such as this, I simply had to make a movie that shows people what can happen when they apply meridian tapping to real life issues. This is how the documentary The Tapping Solution *(formerly known as* Try It On Everything*) came into being.*

The making of the film itself turned out to be a product of tapping in that we, the filmmakers, tapped constantly throughout the shooting of it. I certainly had my doubts about being able to pull the project off! I funded it on credit cards and credit lines and enlisted the help of my younger sister and best friend to create it. None of us had made a movie before or been involved in the film industry so you can imagine the hurdles that came up, both on a practical and a psychological level. We turned to tapping whenever we faced these hurdles and the finished product is a testament to the success of the tapping method.

My intent was to capture the essence and spirit of the tapping process, revealing both its successes and difficulties. Gary Craig's website, www.EmoFree.com, and the contributions of thousands of people around the world who have worked with tapping, has been providing a running conversation about this method for years, one that is open and honest. It documents the hurdles meridian tapping has faced in its development as well as all of its impressive successes. It is because of this conversation that tapping continues to be improved and refined.

The film and its companion book, which you hold in your hand, are a continuation of that ongoing conversation. We have put it out there for you to see, digest, implement, and then add your own contribution to it. We have done our best to be open and honest, presenting both the pluses and minuses of tapping.

I remember that when we decided to conduct the workshop retreat that is the centerpiece of the film, people asked me, "What if it doesn't work? You're flying in ten people from around the U.S. and Canada who face serious emotional and physical challenges − what if they don't get results?" I answered that we would have to show in the movie whatever took place − that's what a documentary is! And we've done just that. Even in instances when we didn't get the results we wished for, such as when Dennis continues to smoke, I made a choice, albeit a difficult one, to include this information in the film. Although there may be thousands of cases around the *world where people have used tapping successfully to quit smoking, in this case that didn't happen and it's important to take a look at the reasons why. We do that in detail in this book.*

Fortunately for us and the world at large, most of the people who came to the workshop event did get astounding results, as documented in the film and further explored in the pages that follow. These people can be admired because they so generously allowed their own personal stories to be shared with thousands of others for the sake of getting the message out, and we thank them deeply.

Of course, there are many things we simply couldn't include in the film. A film cannot explain in detail what meridian tapping actually is, at least not in the way a book can. A film cannot delve deeply into the why and the how of the method, explore its origins and scientific proof, nor can it teach you how to do it for yourself in careful detail.

That is the reason for this book. It has turned out to be the best vehicle to provide the answer the many questions that viewers of the film will inevitably ask. The book can also give the reader a wide variety of true-life stories of people who have applied tapping to numerous challenging issues, and this one also supplies detailed portraits of the ten workshop participants who were filmed in the documentary.

When we looked for an author for this book, we were thrilled to find that a major figure in the meridian tapping world, stress management expert and leading psychologist, Dr. Patricia Carrington, was not only willing to take it on, but was so excited about doing it that she couldn't wait to get started. We knew that Pat had written several well-known books in the stress management field, but were delighted to see the enthusiasm with which she undertook this assignment. Meridian tapping is one of her great loves. In fact she is a pioneer in this technique, having practiced a form of tapping with her clients for over twenty years. She has also created important innovations in tapping, such as the Choices Method, now used by thousands of people worldwide. Pat sees tapping as "the people's method... there for all of us, and literally at our fingertips."

Our film continued the conversation about tapping that had been building online and in workshops and meetings around the world; now this companion book takes that conversation still further. It is my wish that the film, the book, and all the other excellent resources on meridian tapping will make a real difference in your life. However, that will only happen when you try it. Reading books and watching films will set the stage for you, but you must be sure to have a personal experience with tapping. That's the only way you'll unleash its amazing powers and prove its value to yourself.

Tapping can change the way you feel, release pain in your body and help you let go of limiting beliefs, old hurts and traumas in a matter of minutes. Use it! A life of joy, happiness and abundance is waiting for you and it may be just a few "taps" away!

Nicolas Ortner
Creator/Producer of the Film *The Tapping Solution*

Some Words of Thanks

So many people have given of their energy, thought and dedication to make this book possible that I see a panorama of faces before me as I think about it.

Outstanding among these, of course, is Gary Craig, the Founder of Emotional Freedom Techniques (EFT), a leading meridian tapping technique which, as you will see, this book refers to repeatedly.

Gary, as you may know, runs an encyclopedic website, www. EmoFree.com, that contains a carefully compiled, ever-growing collection of articles that chronicle various uses of tapping. His site is a treasure trove of information for anyone interested in learning the subtleties of this technique for their own use, as well as for researchers and historians. The detailed accounts by real EFT users authenticate the method in a powerful manner. Gary also provides a wealth of training materials on DVDs that are a must for any serious student of his method, EFT. The articles archived on his site were contributed by both health care professionals and members of the general public over a period of more than 12 years. It is contributors such as these who have built the foundation upon which meridian tapping techniques rests today. Thanks seems a weak word to use when acknowledging their generously provided help.

To help me accurately present some of the main uses of EFT in this book, Gary Craig has kindly permitted me to reprint (or summarize) here a number of the authentic reports from his site. These reports originally appeared in his newsletter and are reprinted here together with the names of their authors. They can be found on pages 4, 5, 31, 77, 79, 81, 87, 89, 93, 95, 96, 97, 98, 101, 103, 104, 112, 116, 126, 128, 129, 131, 132, 133, 139, 142, and 144 and provide impressive evidence of the enthusiasm and innovativeness of meridian tapping users worldwide. They are testimony to tapping's remarkable usefulness around the globe.

I want to give special thanks, too, to the EFT Masters, that group of highly skilled and trained practitioners originally designated as "Master Practitioners" of EFT by Gary Craig after rigorous testing by him. The original EFT Masters (there will be no others since the training program that graduated them has now been discontinued) now act independently to bring meridian tapping to its highest point of excellence for those interested in its many applications. These original 29 practitioners are in the forefront of meridian tapping education and training worldwide and operate a major website at www.EFTMastersWorldwide.com.

I am also extremely grateful to those who contributed even more directly to the creation of this book through their enlightened help and support: in particular my excellent editor/advisor, Andrew Wolfendon (an articulate tapping advocate as well as a skilled editor), and Nicolas and Jessica Ortner, co-producers of the documentary film *The Tapping Solution*, formerly known as *Try It On Everything*, who have untiringly supplied in-depth information about the participants of the retreat workshop featured in their movie, and who fine-combed the manuscript to assure that it represents meridian tapping in the most authentic and complete manner.

This all brings me to the point where I am deeply grateful that I can now present the finished work to you, and thereby join the rising tide of those who are attempting to spread the word about tapping to the world. My hope is that it helps you in your exploration of this beautiful method.

Patricia Carrington, Ph.D.
Kendall Park, New Jersey

LEGAL DISCLAIMER

Before Reading This Book Please Read This Disclaimer

The information presented in this book, Discover the Power of Meridian Tapping is educational in nature and is provided only as general information. As part of this book, you understand that you will be introduced to a modality called meridian tapping techniques which is a method referred to as a type of "Energy Therapy". To date, meridian tapping has yielded remarkable results for relieving emotional and physical distress, and appears to have promising mental, spiritual, and physical health benefits, but it has yet to be extensively researched by the Western academic, medical, and psychological communities. The prevailing premise is that meridian tapping uses the ancient Chinese meridian system to relieve emotional distress and physiological pain. It is said to balance the energy system with a gentle tapping procedure which stimulates designated meridian end points on the face and body. By reading this book you understand that meridian tapping could be considered experimental and the author and publisher do not know how you will personally respond to meridian tapping and whether meridian tapping will help you with a particular problem.

Due to this experimental nature of meridian tapping, and because it is a relatively new healing approach and the extent of its effectiveness, as well as its risks and benefits are not fully known as yet, you agree to assume and accept full responsibility for any and all risks associated with reading this book and using meridian tapping as a result of reading it. You understand that your choice to use meridian tapping is of your own free will and not subject to any outside pressure. You further understand that if you choose to use meridian tapping, it is possible that emotional or physical sensations or unresolved memories may surface which could be perceived as negative side effects. Emotional material may continue to surface after using meridian tapping, indicating that other issues may need to be addressed. Previously vivid or traumatic memories may fade which could adversely impact your ability to provide detailed legal testimony regarding a traumatic incident.

The information contained in this book, including introducing meridian tapping, is not intended to represent that meridian tapping can be used to diagnose, treat, cure, or prevent any disease or psychological disorder. Meridian tapping is not a substitute for medical or psychological treatment. Consequently, reading the book and using meridian tapping on yourself does not replace health care from medical/psychological professionals. You agree to consult with your health care provider for any specific medical/psychological problems. In addition, you understand that any information contained in the book is not to be considered a recommendation that you stop seeing any of your health care professionals or stop using prescribed medication without consulting with your health care professional, even if after reading the book and using meridian tapping it appears and indicates that such medication or therapy is unnecessary.

Any stories or testimonials presented in this book do not constitute a warranty, guarantee, or prediction regarding the outcome of you as an individual using meridian tapping for any particular issue. While all materials and references to other resources are given in good faith, the accuracy, validity, effectiveness, completeness, or usefulness of any information in this book, cannot be guaranteed. The author and publisher accept no responsibility or liability whatsoever for the use or misuse of the information contained in this book. The author and publisher strongly advise that you seek professional advice as appropriate before implementing any protocol or opinion expressed in this book, including meridian tapping, and before making any health decisions.

By continuing to read this book, you knowingly, voluntarily, and intelligently assume these risks, including any adverse outcome that might result from using meridian tapping, and agree to release, indemnify, hold harmless and defend the author and publisher, and their respective heirs, agents, consultants, and employees from and against any and all claims which you, or your representatives may have for any loss, damage, or injury of any kind or nature arising out of or in connection with reading this book and using meridian tapping. If any court of law rules that any part of this Disclaimer is invalid, the Disclaimer stands as if those parts were struck out.

PLEASE ENJOY THE BOOK AND HAVE FUN WITH TAPPING!

Part 1

The Story of Meridian Tapping

I think we're all looking for something to help us feel better, but in a real way. Tapping isn't just taking a pill, it is something we're engaged in — we're *involved* in this process.*

Carol Look
LCSW, EFT Master, EFT Cert-Honors
Meridian Tapping Expert

To tap is to take responsibility for ourselves.

*Quote from Carol Look from the movie, *The Tapping Solution*.

Chapter 1

Too Good To Be True?

Linda Stotenberg is the owner of a beauty salon in Baltimore. In 1998 her fear of flying had become almost paralyzing. She had been fainting and vomiting during every plane trip. For the previous ten years she had somehow managed to travel but with mounting anxiety on every trip. It was in October of that year that she realized that getting back on a plane would be impossible for her.

That's when she called her good friend Deborah Mitnick whom she knew to be an excellent therapist, and asked her to use a beneficial meridian tapping method on her, known as EFT (Emotional Freedom Techniques). It was reported to combat irrational fears. Deborah must have heard Linda's desperation on the phone, because she agreed to see her right away.

When she arrived at the office, Linda was quickly led through a session of tapping. After they did the full tapping procedure, working for over an hour to root out all her lingering fears, to her astonishment Linda "knew" she could fly again. The next day she got on her plane and had a pleasantly uneventful flight — no fears, no fainting, no vomiting. Since that time Linda has flown with complete ease and thoroughly enjoys it. She credits tapping with giving her back one of the great pleasures in her life — travel.

If that seems too quick and easy an approach to possibly be permanent, consider the report of the Fried family.

A Tapping Way of Life

Stephanie Fried is a Licensed Professional Counselor in New Jersey whose whole family routinely uses tapping as a way of handling life's challenges as they arise. They have used it to help their son feel more confident before Little League games, to eliminate pain or discomfort of an illness or accident for all of them at various times, for helping one of the children handle an impending separation from a best friend and for helping both of them adjust to the death of their much beloved grandfather. If a traumatic accident occurs within the family, the other family members use tapping to help with the shock reaction. Now, whenever something goes wrong, the Fried family automatically asks a family member, "Have you tapped on it?"

If this sounds somewhat "New Age-y" listen to how a prominent athlete has used the meridian tapping method, EFT, and what he has to say about the improvement it made in his game.

Baseball's "EFT Effect"

Pat Ahearne, Australian Baseball League Pitcher of the Year, has publicly stated, "I am so amazed with the effectiveness of EFT that I've made it as important a part of my baseball routine as throwing or running or lifting weights."

Pat was introduced to EFT by Steve Wells, a prominent psychologist in Perth, Australia. They worked together to use EFT to lessen or eliminate the mental emotional barriers preventing Pat from consistently producing his best games as a pitcher. "The results," Pat tells us," were astounding. I had more consistency, better command of my pitches and accomplished more in big games with less effort."

His baseball stats speak for themselves, particularly when we look at the ERA (Earned Run Average), which is the gold standard by which pitchers are measured. Here are Pat's "before" and "after" scores:

	Win-Loss Record	Innings Pitched	Hits Given Up	Earned runs	Walks Given up	Strike-outs	Earned run average
Before EFT	4-2	46	43	17	18	35	3.33
After EFT	3-1	41.3	15	4	7	37	0.87

Pat sums this up by saying, "With EFT I found the edge that raises an athlete from average to elite. I used the technique to capture the MVP of the Perth Heat and the Australian Baseball League Pitcher of the Year Award." Pat is still using EFT extensively.

What does this tell us about EFT? Clearly "something happened" when Pat began using the method that he credits with changing his entire career as an athlete.

Applying Healthy Skepticism

If you are like most newcomers to tapping, at this point you may wonder, "If it really works that well, how come I haven't heard about it before?" That's an obvious question, and the answer lies in the inevitable time lag that occurs when anything of a revolutionary nature is introduced into technology or science. We will talk about that time lag later.

In the meantime, I invite you to be as skeptical as you want. It won't affect the results you get from meridian tapping. If tapping is going to work for you, as it does for over 90% of people who try it, it will work for you regardless of what you think about it. Unless, of course, you are dead set on defeating it and employ strenuous efforts to do so. Such is the power of the mind that you can defeat any treatment if you try hard enough. But with tapping you would have to really try hard!

Here is another one of those "unbelievable tales" of tapping.

Speaking Up with Meridian Tapping

George Edington, M.A., a retired clinical psychologist from Northern New Jersey, had a friend who was so anxious when he had to speak in front of groups that he found himself barely able to talk at all during the important support group meetings he was attending. However, it was critical that he be able to participate in this group. Accordingly, George taught him tapping by having him watch a DVD which I had created and tap along with the film. He then suggested a couple of tapping phrases his friend might use and sent him on his way, instructing him to tap just before the meeting and to excuse himself during the meeting if he felt anxious about speaking, to tap away the fear.

The friend agreed to this plan because he was impressed with the way tapping had already made him feel a lot more comfortable about the meeting. After the meeting he phoned George to tell him that he had tapped as suggested, and that for the first time in his life he had felt no strain whatsoever in front of a group. He now couldn't understand why he had ever thought of public speaking as difficult or tension making.

George's friend needed to remember to tap before each meeting for a while, but eventually he got so used to successfully talking to the group that he no longer needed to do it at all.

Such is the staying power of meridian tapping.

I could go on giving example after example of people in everyday situations who have used tapping to overcome emotional blocks that were hampering their lives. I could also cite hundreds of instances where it has been used to erase the negative effects of major traumas such as natural disasters, war, rape or other life-threatening or demoralizing experiences.

But this is not necessary. You are soon going to experience tapping firsthand and find out what it can do for *you*.

Some Common Reasons for Resisting Tapping

Now let's look briefly at some of the more common reasons people hesitate to try a new technique such as meridian tapping and see whether any of these might apply to you:

- Do you suspect that any treatment that could address your problem will involve digging up painful feelings and memories and then revealing them to someone else? You may be reluctant to face that emotional hurdle.

- Have you tried many treatments in the past that failed and are unwilling to risk failing once again? If none of these well-known methods could help you, what makes you think that a little known and seemingly illogical method derived from acupuncture could work? You may not want to try and fail once more.

- After many a futile attempt to overcome a longstanding mental/emotional issue, you may have decided the issue is so deeply engrained that it will require a lot of work to resolve. You may have put off that work for another day, or have simply been unable to identify what that "work" should be.

- You may have finally decided, after repeated unsuccessful attempts to change, that this is "just the way I am" and learned to settle for a diminished life.

And Now the Bold Promises of Meridian Tapping...

Meridian tapping is a remarkably simple and powerful self-administered technique. You can apply it to yourself at any time, or use it under the guidance of a trained Practitioner.

Tapping:
- Often works where nothing else has.
- Is gentle and easy.
- Has effects that are almost always lasting.
- Can be used in privacy without any need to disclose your personal issues to anyone.
- Can also be used with the help of an experienced meridian tapping therapist in the case of a particularly difficult or engrained problem if you wish — this can lessen the time and effort involved in traditional psychotherapy.

Of course, meridian tapping is not 100% effective in all cases in the same way that pharmaceuticals or any other therapeutic interventions are not effective in all instances. Nor does it always create long-term results in a single session. But it *has* proven so effective at quickly and permanently altering negative emotions, troubling thoughts, destructive behavior patterns and a long list of psychological and even physical symptoms that even the skeptical scientific community is beginning to sit up and take notice, although they may grumble a bit. Meridian tapping is proving to be one of the most potent and simple therapeutic interventions ever introduced. Extensive clinical practice and research is bearing this out.

Just Another "Quick Fix"?

Although most of us are reluctant to believe that serious, deep-seated psychological issues can be alleviated with a quick, simple treatment, let's look at medicine for a moment. There are many illnesses and debilitating conditions that people once believed had to be suffered for months, years, or lifetimes. Perhaps some of the most unbearable symptoms of these illnesses could be palliated, but hoping to defeat the disease itself was unimaginable. Then one day — presto! — science discovers a cure. How? By learning to treat the problem in an entirely new way. The disease is then quickly eliminated or becomes a minor blip on our radar screens. Usually this has involved identifying the true origin of the problem and treating it at its source.

The discovery that stress and allergic reactions create many disorders, for example, has allowed us to treat certain symptoms with astounding simplicity and effectiveness. We don't complain about "quick fixes" when the mere removal of a down pillow or a house plant from our environment clears up a ten-year sore throat. We don't cry "foul" when a long overdue confrontation with our boss clears up a problem and causes our migraines to cease. On the contrary, we are delighted that such a fast, painless and effective solution is available.

Today the healing professions are learning, or perhaps we should say, re-learning, that life is basically an "energetic"

The electrical system in the body is more intricate than anything in a house. It would make the electrical system in a super computer look like an absolute toy. And we really don't understand much about it!*

Bob Proctor
Success Mentor
Featured in "The Secret"

Tapping works to remove blockages in the human energy system, making meridian tapping a powerful healing tool.

*Quote from Bob Proctor from the movie, *The Tapping Solution*.

phenomenon. Emotions are actually specific forms of energy, just as the electric current that sizzles your microwave popcorn is a form of energy. As energy, emotions can be treated directly and simply. This is a radical new approach for mainstream psychology and medicine.

Meridian tapping does an end-run around traditional, long-term therapies by applying (or helping traditional approaches to apply) treatment to the actual blockages which are perhaps not surprisingly located in the mind/body's energy system. Change the energy pattern and you change the emotion. It is really that simple and direct.

So how was meridian tapping developed, and why? These important questions deserve a chapter of their own.

Chapter 2

It's All About Energy

1209 B.C. A tiny farming village in China.

A young woman hunches over a failing bean plant. She taps on a stem here, gently pinches a leaf there, tries to coax a better flow of life energy or *Qi* (pronounced chee) to the pods. Suddenly she cries out in pain and falls to her knees. A passing villager hears her shriek and rushes to investigate. He finds her doubled over writhing with pain, in the dirt. She is gripping her abdomen and grimacing.

"Wait!" he shouts at her, and dashes off to enlist the aid of a neighboring farmer. This is the third time in as many days that this woman has fallen to the ground in pain. Together, the men carry her to the pounded-dirt walls of the nearby town. She is taken to the physician's house immediately.

The elderly healer instructs her to sit up before him. He holds her head in his hands and studies the shape and position of her tongue. He listens to her breath, sniffs it, appraises its temperature. He tests her heartbeat on several points on her body. He asks her about recent chills and fever, her appetite, her menses, her sleep patterns. He presses her flesh in various parts of her body, testing for tender spots.

At last, after a long and thoughtful pause, he opens an ornate box filled with delicate needles, all in rows. With a creased brow and a steady hand, he begins carefully inserting them, one by one, into the skin of her *face*…

The woman sighs as her gut releases its tight clench of pain. She is starting to feel relief…

Her future treatment will consist of further visits and more strategically placed needles, and she may be asked to drink healing teas between times. The physician will be gradually coaxing the vital *qi* energy back into its proper path (i.e. restoring its active circuits) so that it now flows unobstructed — the precondition for healing to take place. This is the same process the woman used with the bean plant. Both she and the physician know how to redirect the flow of energy in living systems. It is the ancient Chinese people's way of healing, a wisdom available to everyone, no matter what their station in life or physical condition.

2008 A.D. A Suburb of Boston in the United States

A middle-aged man sits in a psychologist's waiting room, his leg jittering nervously up and down. He grabs a magazine, glances at the cover story about some starlet's latest rehab romance, but the words make no sense today. He tosses the magazine down, takes a long, deep breath.

What am I doing here, he asks himself. He stands up, paces the floor, decides that he is going to head for the nearest coffee shop instead. He is inches from a clean getaway when the door to the inner office opens and the psychologist beckons him in.

"You probably can't help me," he announces before even finding his seat. The man explains to the psychologist that he has developed an intense fear of riding in automobiles. This fear is particularly acute when he attempts to drive past a certain major intersection where he has had not one, but *two* car accidents in recent months. The second accident occurred while he was trying to "psych" himself up in order to overcome his fear and resistance following the first accident. Now he finds himself having a hard time driving anywhere, but utterly incapable of driving through the ill-fated intersection. This is no small inconvenience — it is the main road junction in town.

The man has learned to detour around the troublesome site, a detour that takes him about five miles out of his way every day, going to and from work. This week, however, the *detour* road has gone under construction and will be closed to through traffic for a period of many weeks. The only way to avoid this trouble spot will now be a route that will require him to drive a full twenty five minutes out of his way. He has decided that this is ridiculous and he needs to face the problem head on.

He explains to the psychologist that he doesn't have the time, money or interest to pursue long-term psychotherapy.

"I'm going to ask you to consider a technique that has proven to be extremely effective in eliminating fears such as you describe," the psychologist tells him. "It's called meridian tapping. I must warn you: it may seem a little strange to you because it requires tapping on your face and upper body. Are you willing to try it, anyway?"

He says yes.

She begins by asking him to rate his general fear of driving on a scale of one to ten, as he feels the fear *right now*, with ten being as anxious as he can imagine being.

"Eight," he replies without hesitation.

She then instructs him to repeat the sentence, "Even though I have this fear of riding in a car, I deeply and completely accept myself." The man shoots her a dubious look, but utters the given words.

Soon the psychologist is leading him through a somewhat mysterious ritual that involves making repeated affirmations while *tapping* his body at key locations: the inner side of the eyebrow, under the nose, beneath the armpit, and so forth

The process takes only a few minutes, after which the psychologist again asks her new patient to rate his general anxiety about driving. The man calmly says , "Well, it's actually pretty much gone. It's down to a 2" and he casts a suspicious glance at her, as if she is a stage magician who has somehow gotten hold of his wallet.

She then asks him to rate his fear about the intersection in particular. The fear of that single location is still registering pretty high, so she asks him to describe aloud his second and most traumatizing car accident. Each time during the story that the man *begins* to feel fearful at all — that is, each time he uncovers a new *Aspect* of the fear (see Chapter 7 for more on "*Aspects*") — the psychologist asks him to tap his way past it. She encourages him to use expressions such as:

"Even though I am afraid to drive through the
     intersection…"

"Even though I am afraid I will be hit again…"

"Even though I feel helpless to prevent being hit by a car…
     I deeply and completely accept myself."

She asks him to conclude by tapping to the statement, "Even
though I have this fear of driving through the intersection… I
choose to know that the danger is over and I'm safe now."

When the process is finished, she asks him again to describe his
fear. The man states that he believes he can now drive through
the problem intersection without difficulty

However, as the saying goes, the proof of the pudding is in
the eating. The man calmly drives directly to work the following
day, negotiating the intersection without a hitch. Even when he
hears the squeal of fast-braking tires nearby, he remains peaceful
and confident. In this particular instance he needs no further
sessions with the psychologist. Tapping has done it's job and he
now can use it, any time he wants to, for himself.

What common thread do these two stories share?

It's All About "Energy"

If you have read anything at all about acupuncture, you
probably know it is based on the concept of a flow of a
special sort of *vital energy* throughout the body. According to
Traditional Chinese Medicine (TCM) this energy, or *qi*, flows
through the body along certain invisible pathways called
Meridians. You probably also know that according to TCM all
things living possess both *yin* qualities and *yang* qualities. Yin
is cold, dark, "negative," and passive. Yang is warm, light,
"positive" and active. Acupuncturists believe that illnesses are
a result of imbalances in our yin and our yang aspects, caused
by a disruption in the normal flow of *qi* throughout the living
system. In effect, some of the body's energy circuits have been
short-circuited. Stated in one sentence, the premise behind
acupuncture might be summed up as: *The cause of pain and illness
is a **disruption** in the body's energy system.*

The insertion of needles into strategic points on the skin helps to reestablish harmony within the system by adjusting the flow of *qi* to correct troublesome disruptions.

Because no standard measuring instrument as yet exists (one will probably soon be created) that can demonstrate the existence of these meridian pathways in a manner fully acceptable to "hard science," the meridian theory on which acupuncture is based can sound quaint and folktale-esque to the modern scientific mind. In fact, it would be easy for us in the modern world to dismiss acupuncture entirely, except for one stubborn and annoying fact.

It works.

Acupuncture is used successfully in both the East and West to treat a wide range of ailments, including headaches, nausea, depression, sinus infections, muscle sprains, skin conditions and numerous other distressing conditions. Pain management is a major application in hospitals in both the East and West, even those that otherwise operate conservatively. Western visitors to China have been stunned to see open heart surgery performed on smiling, wide-awake patients whose only anesthesia is a cluster of thin needles in the ear. Many other anesthetic applications of acupuncture are now being used in hospitals in the United States and elsewhere.

Because acupuncture does not mesh with our modern Western view of anatomy and physiology, however, we are quick to attribute its positive results to "placebo" effects — it works because patients *want* it to work. But then, how do we explain its effectiveness on animals? Acupuncture is now being adopted more and more by veterinary medicine in many countries throughout the world. Increasingly, veterinarians are using tiny needles to treat dogs, cats, horses, and other creatures for problems such as chronic pain and arthritic stiffness, when other methods fail. Presumably, race horses and show dogs don't have belief systems and hidden agendas. Something else must be at work here.

To shed light on this mystery, let's look at how medicine presently conceives of the human body. Is the ancient idea of the body as a system of energy pathways really so inconsistent with modern views? If the concept of vital energy is so alien to us, why then do we hook up patients to electronic sensors to monitor their "life-force"? Why is a flat line on an ECG machine (meaning "no electrical activity") such a disturbing thing to see in a hospital room? And why do we jump-start the hearts of fellow human beings with scary-looking *electric* paddles?

The fact is, the human body — life itself — can easily be seen as an elaborate *energy system*. What is a nerve impulse but a form of energy known as electricity traveling along a pathway? What is an ECG or an EEG but the measure of the electrical activity (the energy) of the heart and brain? Every organ and body system seems to have its corresponding energy field and pathways. U.S. Army tests have measured the electromagnetic field of the human heart as it extends up to eight feet outside of the body. These fields and currents are measurable, tangible. Without the continuous flow of life energy through the body, there is no life.

The dreaded flat line on the ECG.

The fact is that energy *is* life. Life *is* energy. They are one and the same.

This is consistent with what we are finding to be true for the rest of nature. One of the great discoveries of the 20th Century is that *everything* in the observable universe is made up, essentially, of energy. Einstein taught us that matter and energy are interchangeable — ultimately they are one and the same thing. Matter, thought waves, water, radio waves, behaviors such as laughter, or emotions such as sadness are really not different *things*, but may be different *arrangements* of something far more subtle and essential. Matter is now seen by quantum physicists as really wave energy "locked" in a particular form by our act of observation. It is energy that is "frozen" as we experience it because our senses are designed to perceive it to be that way.

In the modern world most of us are still mesmerized by the tangible and visible. Despite a century of science that has dethroned matter as the ruling monarch of reality, we still cling to the old model of the world that Sir Isaac Newton embraced — a world of colliding billiard balls causing an endless physical chain of actions and reactions that seem to continue to infinity.

We still see *things* as more real and more worthy of attention than energy. We are in love with the dense, the thick, the heavy, the *visible*.

Naturally, this determines our views of health and medicine. We tend to identify organs, bones and chemicals as our primary targets when practicing medicine. Human energy is seen as little more than an inconvenient discharge given off by the "real stuff".

But what is it that *animates* our bones and muscles? What is the "ghost in the machine" that separates a living, breathing human being from a medical school cadaver? Isn't this *invisible, energetic* aspect of who we are worthy of at least as much attention as the nuts and bolts that we can see and touch? Isn't the TV *show* at least as interesting as the TV *set*? Isn't that which defines us as alive at least as important as that which accompanies us beyond the physical grave — our bones, hair and teeth?

Fortunately, the answer is shifting to "yes." The old model is changing. In recent years experimental studies and well-documented medical cases have forced us to acknowledge some telling challenges to so-called "hard" science. For example:

- A landmark study of 393 hospitalized post-surgery cardiac patients conducted by Randolph Byrd in 1988 showed that prayer directed at those patients (unbeknownst to the patients and at a distance) resulted in significantly faster and more complete recovery in those patients prayed for versus those who were not.

- In research conducted in 1980 by Jeanne Achterberg, subjects were able to increase the production of specific types of white blood cells (T-cells and neutrophils) by using visualization techniques and nothing else.

- In 1974, Robert Ader fed a group of lab rats an immunosuppressive drug mixed with sweet-tasting saccharin. He then switched to saccharin only and was amazed to discover that the rats continued to suffer immune system deficiency. By simple conditioning he had turned a harmless chemical into poison. Mind over matter, even in rats.

- In the 1980s Herbert Benson conducted a series of studies of monks in the Himalayas, who, by practicing a yogic technique known as *Tum-mo*, are able to raise and lower their own body temperature at will. Monks sitting in a 40-degree room and wrapped in cold, wet towels (conditions ideal for developing hypothermia) were able to dry the towels with their body heat, actually making them emit steam.

One could fill a book with "new" discoveries and baffling experiments such as these. What they share in common is that they debunk the myth of material things as the overriding influences in our lives and suggest that subtle and invisible energy is a key factor in the management, growth and support of life. "Soft" science may finally be fusing with hard science.

There could be some unexpected consequences to this shift. We'll now have a look at these as they are illustrated by various cases in which tapping has been used.

Chapter 3

Science Faces a Revolution

Scientific models change with hesitation and slowly, but they *do* change.

Today, we are seeing the first of the new "energy sciences". In biology, for example, one such exciting development is the science of *epigenetics,* developed by cell biologist Bruce Lipton and elaborated brilliantly by Dawson Church in *The Genie in Your Genes.* In his book, Church points out that science is finally beginning to recognize that the mere existence of DNA by itself, *inactivated*, is no more than unrealized potential. It does not, and cannot, orchestrate the unfolding of a biological organism.

Apparently the *expression* of genes is as crucial as their existence. And that expression is controlled, to a large extent, by the *energetic* choices we make — thoughts, emotions, beliefs, decisions — mere "soft" stuff in the eyes of mainstream science.

Genes, Church points out, can be compared to individual musicians and their instruments in a symphony orchestra. Without the introduction of intelligent energy, the instruments just sit there, un-plucked and un-strummed in the hands of musicians who are seemingly frozen in place. It is the *conductor* who coaxes the various musicians and their instruments to express a specific melody. The conductor tells the trumpeter when to play a C-sharp and when to stay silent. The conductor calls the all-important tune. Without the conductor there would be no music, just chaotic sound, or silence.

Similarly, when it comes to genes, the "conductor" is crucial.

And that conductor is *us* — our consciousness, our emotions, the kinds of energy we call upon in our lives. It turns out that *we* can control the *expression* of our genes by the way we live and the choices we make. Beliefs, spiritual practices, attitudes, intentions, and the moods we choose to cultivate all have a demonstrable effect on the expression of our "hard" genetic code. The energies of love and nurturance literally unlock different genes and, consequently, build different kinds of organisms than do the energies of fear and neglect. It is no longer scientifically correct to say, "It's all in the DNA." It's in the DNA, yes, but even more so, it's in the way genes are selectively expressed (or selectively *sup*pressed) through the "soft" energetic choices we make. It is we who run the show.

Psychology Enters the Scene

Psychology has begun to respond to this human energy movement. The relatively new field of Energy Psychology recognizes that we are, first and foremost, *energetic* beings. It looks at energy centers, energy pathways, and bio-fields as vital players in human psychology. It attempts to address stubborn psychological issues by dealing with the bio-energy that is literally *causing* the felt emotional state.

After all, what is an emotion but a form of energy being expressed? If that energy can be re-routed, dispersed or re-shaped, the emotional state will consequently change—directly and immediately, as though we had thrown a switch — which in a sense we have…

While traditional talk therapy can be beneficial in helping us trace the origins of our energy disruptions — and this can be very important — it is the disruption in the *energy field* itself that is immediately responsible for the negative emotions we experience. Energy psychologists are now attempting to treat energy patterns directly. When this is accomplished successfully, as it often is with meridian tapping, remarkable-seeming "miracles" frequently happen. Phobias and self-destructive thinking patterns will often permanently disappear after only one, or a few short treatment sessions. How can this possibly be?

What Is This Tapping All About?

Meridian tapping techniques are often referred to simply as "tapping" for reasons that will soon become obvious. They are self-administered techniques that can be done either alone or under the supervision of a trained meridian tapping therapist in order to relieve negative emotional patterns. If we were to state its underlying premise in one sentence, we would offer a corollary of the statement made earlier about acupuncture: *All negative emotions are a result of a disruption in the body's energy system.*

Does this mean that if a ten ton truck were to run us down in the street so that we suffered severe injury, shock, and terror, that the emotional trauma we would be experiencing would be due merely to a reaction of our energy system to being thrown out of kilter and would have nothing to do with the external impact — the ten ton truck?

Of course not! The physical injury caused by the truck would be very real and the consequent emotional shock totally normal, but what we know now that we didn't before is that something psychologists call an "intervening variable" is at work in this situation. A "middleman" of sorts seems to operate in the fraction of a millisecond between the physical impact and the resultant emotional/bodily response, and this makes it very difficult and sometimes impossible for the body and mind to recover from the accident. That middleman is the immediate (and in the case of the truck's impact, extreme) *disruption* that occurs in our body's energy system as the result of the impact.

When an assault on our physical or emotional integrity occurs, whether this attack is physical or verbal or a result of our own inner fears and frightening self-talk, it immediately throws a STOP switch that can cause massive disruption of the energy system and even result in a form of energetic chaos. It is that disruption, that sudden blockage of our normal healthy energy flow, that makes recovery from a trauma so difficult and sometimes impossible. The disturbing fact is that until this energy blockage is removed and a healthy balance of energy within the body restored, there can be no full and permanent healing from the shock. The body/mind continues to react as though the assault on us is *still going on*.

This means that no matter how much we *talk* about a trauma, or how clearly we come to *understand* what happened to us and why (although all of this certainly helps) it is not until the *energy disruption itself* is addressed that the *Qi* energy can again flow smoothly. Without a rebalancing of the energy system there cannot be complete healing. We may feel better from talking, but if the blockage has not been completely removed from our energy system, much residual disturbance will remain and even a minor occurrence may set off the traumatic reaction once again

This is why a traumatic event can still be damaging or even crippling many decades after it occurred. Its effect may in fact persist for an entire lifetime if the energy disruption caused by that event has not been corrected. And that is why, when the energy system is handled directly as it is in meridian tapping, a sudden and seemingly miraculous "healing" can occur as the normal flow of energy reestablishes itself.

What Energy Intervention Is All About

The new Energy Therapies can often be startlingly rapid and effective. Only when there are numerous repeated traumas to be set right, involving hundreds and sometimes thousands of disrupted energy pathways, does an Energy Psychology treatment require considerable time and persistence — and even then it has a better chance of success than talking about the trauma alone. The combination of the two approaches — talking therapy and meridian tapping — is therefore immensely powerful. It can blast through energy blockages to effect a healing on all levels.

Tapping is, however, deceptively simple. On the surface, at least in the short version most commonly practiced today, it involves nothing more complicated than repeating custom-made verbal affirmations and tapping repeatedly on specific key locations on the body. That's all there is to it — on the surface. Tapping and affirming.

This entire process takes only a few minutes if we are dealing with a single-*Aspect* problem, as we often are. And it takes an incomparably shorter time than any other therapy previously used, even if we are dealing with multiple *Aspects* of the same problem and have to address each of these separately over time. In terms of rapidity and sheer effectiveness, tapping is a true therapeutic breakthrough.

The amazing speed with which it can work is of course due to the fact that unblocking an impedance in an energy pathway is like throwing a switch to restore current to an entire office building — all the lights go on at once and in a fraction of a second. It is not at all uncommon to see lifelong phobias disappear after a single meridian tapping treatment, or to see them disappear after a few tapping sessions when a more complicated series of blockages is involved. If numerous disruptions in the energy system have occurred in complex instances due to many repeated traumas, it may require a prolonged series of meridian tapping treatments to entirely clear the problem, and occasionally, a series of major traumas can never be completely healed, even with tapping, but even at its least effective in extremely complex cases, meridian tapping is still light years ahead of previous therapies in its high level of effectiveness. It often works where nothing else has.

The best way to understand how tapping really works, of course, is to try it for yourself and you will have a chance to do this in Chapter 6. We will now look at how this unusual treatment came about. It is a very interesting story.

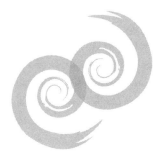

Chapter 4

Tapping's Family Tree

To understand the "pedigree" of meridian tapping, let's go back to acupuncture for a moment. Meridian tapping and acupuncture share a common heritage. They both proceed from the concept that energy flows along precise pathways, or meridians, in the body.

Acupuncture, though, was not designed to treat emotional problems, only physical ones. Although it may be used to relax a patient or to relieve severe anxiety when this is specifically requested, acupuncture does not have a systematic way of addressing emotional problems.

Meridian tapping fills this void. For that reason it is often called "emotional acupuncture." Like most important treatment techniques, it grew in stages and has been refined over the years.

One of the major steps that led to the development of meridian tapping was a discovery by Dr. George Goodheart, a leading U.S. chiropractor. Goodheart found to his surprise that he could achieve the same beneficial results of acupuncture without using the dreaded needle. By simply applying pressure or tapping on identified acupuncture points, his patients were finding relief from a multitude of symptoms. *Stimulating* the acupuncture points (rather than piercing them with sharp objects!) was a much more accessible method for many people, as it was completely non-invasive.

An Australian psychiatrist, John Diamond, M.D., then took this discovery a step further. Diamond began using verbal *affirmations* as the patient was stimulating the acupuncture points. This was a major step forward as it introduced a psychological tool into the process and showed promising results. But still the treatment method lacked a cohesive "engine" to drive it forward with real effectiveness. That engine was to be supplied by Dr. Roger Callahan, an American psychologist specializing in anxiety disorders.

The Callahan Contribution

Dr. Callahan had been studying the meridian energy system for some time, in addition to traditional approaches to medicine and psychiatry. But, as is often the case with great discoveries, it was an "accident" in his office that unlocked the precise key that brought about the development of meridian tapping.

Callahan had been working for over two years with "Mary," a patient who had such an overwhelming fear of water that she could not even get into a bathtub without triggering an anxiety attack. Although Callahan had tried a multitude of anti-anxiety techniques with her, the progress had been slow and discouraging. Mary couldn't even go *near* the swimming pool on the grounds of his office, or allow water to touch her body, without panicking.

One day Mary told Dr. Callahan, for the first time, that her fearful feeling was located specifically in her stomach. Callahan knew about an acupuncture point located directly beneath the eye that is traditionally linked to the stomach meridian. He asked Mary to tap on that point, in hopes that it might balance a possible disturbance in her meridian energy system and lessen her stomach symptoms. He had no idea it would have profound implications for the future of his practice and for psychology as a whole.

Mary dutifully tapped under her eye, as instructed, and a totally unexpected thing happened. Instead of merely experiencing relief from her stomach symptoms, she announced that her lifelong fear of water was suddenly gone! It had simply vanished. Callahan was stunned to watch her rise from her chair and run outside toward the swimming pool. Because he knew she couldn't swim, he ran after her, concerned for her safety. When she reached the pool, she began splashing water on her face and laughing, completely at ease. Her fear of water had simply been *erased* (permanently, as it turned out).

This was surprising, to say the least. Callahan had stumbled upon a key discovery upon which the future of meridian tapping would later be based, namely that if a person is focusing on a specific fear at the time they tap, that fear can be removed, often permanently. He decided to explore the possibility of using strategic tapping to treat other phobias as well. While not all phobias disappeared as rapidly as Mary's had, some did. A new technology based on tapping and affirming had been born.

Dr. Callahan then developed his discovery into a complete system. He concluded that there was a correct tapping *sequence* for every emotional issue, and that this could be determined for each individual through the use of muscle testing. He called these tapping sequences "algorithms" and his treatment became known as Thought Field Therapy, or TFT.

Dr. Callahan's work was brilliant and groundbreaking and produced many astonishing "cures." It did, however, have some practical drawbacks that prevented it from being more widely practiced. First of all, the muscle testing used to calibrate the treatment was cumbersome and could only be performed by a professional trained in kinesiology, which meant that patients could not perform the procedure independently. Second, the system was complex and difficult to master, as different algorithms were required for each one of the numerous disorders studied.

The Next Stage is Launched

Some practitioners of TFT began to wonder if there was a way to simplify and standardize the process. Was it possible, perhaps, to create a single tapping sequence that could work in all cases? What if the patient could "cover the waterfront" with each tapping session, hitting *all* of the major anti-anxiety acupuncture points every single time? Wouldn't a global treatment routine eliminate the need for the cumbersome individualized algorithms?

Here is where I enter the picture as a clinical psychologist who was at that time teaching at Princeton University, and Gary Craig, an engineer and personal performance coach who had been one of Roger Callahan's star pupils, become a major player in the meridian tapping story. Neither Gary nor I knew of each other and neither of us had heard of the other's attempts to explore this possibility, but at almost the same time we both arrived at an identical conclusion, namely that a single-algorithm tapping method might be *just as effective* as the more elaborate, multiple procedures of TFT.

By 1988, I had developed a simplified tapping technique based on Callahan's TFT, which I called "Acutap." Skipping the diagnostic procedure entirely, I simply asked people to tap on the acupuncture end-points used by Callahan each time they did a round of tapping. Using this method, I was able to help my clients in ways that had never been possible before and Acutap revolutionized my practice as a clinical psychologist.

Gary Craig, meanwhile, was developing his own single-algorithm method which he called "Emotional Freedom Techniques (EFT)" to distinguish it from TFT. As soon as I tried EFT, I recognized that is possessed some excellent features that Acutap did not. I immediately began using Craig's EFT method instead of Acutap, and then added a number of refinements to this tapping method such as my Choices Method, now a major tapping technique of its own. Since the mid-1990s it has been the mainstay of my psychological practice. My writings and professional life now center around this remarkable method.

The Growth of Meridian Tapping

Meridian tapping is now the most influential and widely known Energy Psychology method in the world, and Gary's authority in the field is followed closely by the 29 EFT practitioners who were designated by him as "EFT Masters" after meeting the rigorous requirements of his training program (I am privileged to be one of these Masters!). Although Gary has formally ended the Masters Training Program which granted us this honor and there will be no designated EFT Masters after us, we continue to train other practitioners in meridian tapping and this method is spreading rapidly.

By now, through his classic DVDs, manual and extremely popular newsletter, Gary has brought EFT to the attention of millions of people worldwide. I have meanwhile have gone on to develop the Choices Method, an advanced version of meridian tapping which is now included in the repertoire of most practitioners. It can be learned by means of the Choices Manual, Gary's DVD of my Choices Workshop, and other educational materials.

All evidence suggests that meridian tapping may soon transform psychological treatment for emotional problems once believed to be treatable only by lengthy and partially-effective procedures. The journey of over 50 years from acupuncture to meridian tapping has resulted in meridian-based treatments for emotional issues now gaining familiarity and acceptance around the world.

We will now explore the research in this area — unless of course you want to start learning to tap immediately, in which case you can go directly to Chapter 6 without delay!

Chapter 5

A Look at the Proof

The question, of course, is "Does meridian tapping *really* work?" Or are its results merely due to a vivid imagination on the part of those who try it and their *wish* to have it work"?

The answer is clear. The research is coming in and it's telling us that tapping represents a genuine advance in the psychological and medical fields. Quantifiable, measurable results are showing up, and, equally important, they are *holding* up, around the world.

I'm going to give you a quick summary of some of the recent studies that have been done. If you are interested in reading about them in more detail and want to see the latest up-to-date information, I suggest you visit the Resource section of my website, www.TappingCentral.com.

Here's the short version.

The First Major Study

The first major laboratory research on meridian tapping is the well-known Wells Study, reported in *The Journal of Clinical Psychology* in 2003. A team of Australian researchers headed by psychologist Steve Wells, tested the EFT form of tapping against a deep-breathing technique as a treatment for fears/phobias of small creatures such as rats and cockroaches. They wanted to know whether EFT would be effective in delivering immediate benefits to the participants, and they wanted to answer the all-important question of whether any benefits gained through EFT would hold up over time.

The results were eye-opening. EFT proved to be far more effective than the comparison technique in four out of five measures (for the fifth measure, pulse-rate, there was no statistical difference). But perhaps the most significant revelation of this study was that when the subjects were re-tested 6 to 9 months later, the gains achieved through EFT had held up much more strongly than those achieved by the comparison method. And that was after these subjects had had only a single 30-minute EFT session and no intervening treatments!

Another Team Takes It Further

Spurred by Wells' impressive results, a second team of scientists, led by Dr Harvey Baker in New York, decided to try to replicate the Wells Study. They added a few new twists. The comparison method they used was called the Supportive Interview and made use of a techniques commonly employed in talk therapy. They also added a third, "control" group of subjects who were present in the lab but received no treatment at all. Finally, they stretched the total time period of the study to 1.38 years.

Their results showed that although the initial beneficial effects of EFT shrunk a bit over time, they had not *disappeared* by the follow-up retesting over a year later. And, as with the Wells study, the subjects had received no further treatment during the interim.

Both the Baker-Siegel research and the Wells study demonstrate that meridian tapping has not only immediate benefits but long-term potency.

A Study of EFT and Post-Traumatic Stress

In another EFT study, published in *The Journal of Subtle Energies & Energy Medicine*, a Canadian research team studied 9 victims of motor vehicle accidents who had been experiencing severe post-traumatic stress symptoms. These subjects were given a battery of tests, both psychological and neurophysiological, before and after learning meridian tapping. Before tapping, they reported average distress ratings of 8.3 on a 0 to 10-point scale of intensity when thinking about their accidents. Their brain waves generally corresponded with their psychological tests. After they had been treated with EFT, however, their average intensity rating had come down to 2.5, an extremely significant change. Bottom line—all 9 accident victims showed positive change after EFT. They were then given a "homework assignment" to continue with their therapeutic tapping on a specific, regular schedule.

After a period of 70 to 160 days, all were re-tested and an interesting development showed up in both the brainwave patterns and the results of the psychological questionnaires. For 5 of the 9 participants the positive changes had held up excellently, but for 4 of these subjects they had not. This study, unfortunately, did not look at how well the participants had complied with their home-treatment assignment, so that may well have been the deciding factor. Still, 5 out of 9 subjects showing long-term positive results for a condition as serious as post traumatic stress is extremely encouraging and convincing.

Tapping's Use for Epilepsy

In another study, Dr. Paul Swingle used EFT as a treatment for 25 preschool children who were diagnosed with epilepsy and for whom anti-seizure medication was risky because of their age. The results were striking. Dr. Swingle found substantial reductions in seizure frequency, as well as extensive clinical improvement in the children's EEG readings, after only two weeks of daily in-home EFT treatment.

A Six-Month Study of Over 100 EFT Users

More recently a large-group study, initiated by psychologist Jack Rowe, published in the *Counseling & Clinical Psychology Journal*, was conducted with participants at an EFT conference led by Gary Craig. Over a hundred attendees took the SCL 90-R, a highly respected measure of psychological distress, on five different occasions: one month before the workshop commenced; at the beginning of the workshop: at the end of the workshop: and then again one month, and six months after the workshop.

The results showed a highly significant decrease in distress from pre-workshop to immediately after the workshop. Six months later, the gains made at the workshop were still holding up strongly, although some diminishment of intensity was recorded, as might be expected.

Other less formal studies continue to feed us important information and clues as to EFT's value.

Meridian Tapping Surprisingly Improves Eyesight!

Dr. Carol Look, a prominent meridian tapping expert and one of the founding EFT Masters, conducted an experiment online that showed a marked improvement in subjects' *eyesight* when they had been systematically tapping on unrelated emotions such as fear, anger, guilt, and others. *Nearly 75%* of participants reported visual improvement over the course of the study. Tapping on anger, interestingly enough, seemed to produce the strongest results.

Tapping Calms Dental Fears

Dr. Graham Temple, a dentist and professionally-trained meridian tapping practitioner in the UK, conducted his own study on the effects of EFT on highly anxious dental patients. Seventy-two percent of patients—almost three out of four—achieved a level of comfort and a feeling of control that allowed them to cope well with the dental work that followed.

And here's the "Kicker"

In a sports-related "informal" study done by Sam Smith of Australia, EFT was used on participants in a rugby-kicking competition. The subjects were asked to take free kicks from various distances before and after learning EFT. There was an overall improvement in performance of 80.7% after EFT was applied. Gary Craig, whose web site reports this study in detail, points out that part of this improvement could be attributed to getting better with practice. But, as a very experienced athlete himself, he estimates that only 10% to 20% of the improvement seen here could be attributed to a "practice effect."

We could look at many more studies that have shown EFT's effectiveness in a variety of areas, and we will soon be seeing published studies showing similar effectiveness for other variants of meridian tapping. EFT was the first and obvious choice of the researchers because it had already been studied by others, a prerequisite for many research projects. Other forms of meridian tapping will undoubtably be the subjects of research as the method spreads worldwide.

But now you get a chance to experience tapping firsthand.

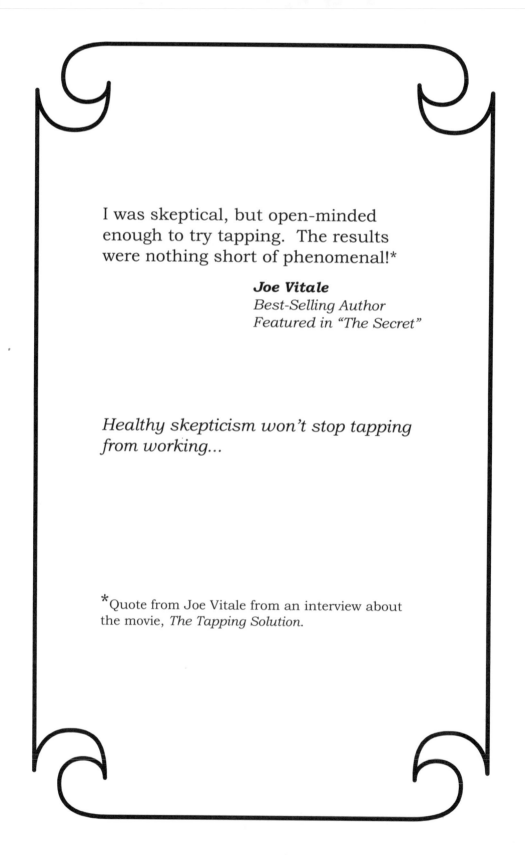

I was skeptical, but open-minded enough to try tapping. The results were nothing short of phenomenal!*

Joe Vitale
Best-Selling Author
Featured in "The Secret"

Healthy skepticism won't stop tapping from working...

*Quote from Joe Vitale from an interview about the movie, *The Tapping Solution*.

Part 2

Learning Meridian Tapping

What I often say to clients is, "You know what? I have this little tapping technique that I think might be really helpful here.

It might seem a little strange, but if you're willing to play along and work with me, let's just give it a try and see what happens.*

Cheryl Richardson
Personal Coaching Pioneer
Best-Selling Author

Tapping may seem awkward at first, but it is rooted in a natural way of using our hands to comfort ourselves.

*Quote from Cheryl Richardson from the movie, *The Tapping Solution.*

Chapter 6

Basic Steps
(the 'How to' Chapter)

> **IMPORTANT NOTICE**
>
> *This method of stress management is easily mastered by most people in a short period of time, but it is not a form of psychotherapy. People who have medical or emotional problems that require professional attention, should use this program as they would any other stress relief method, under the supervision of their physician or other qualified health professional.*

By the time you finish this chapter, you will have learned all the basics of meridian tapping and have had a chance to apply it to an issue of your own. You will have gotten hands-on experience with tapping which will allow you to and can then go on to explore this method further to master its subtleties. Or, you may decide to stop at this point and apply tapping in your own way and find this very satisfactory. Either way, you are in for an adventure, and quite possibly for some surprises.

For best results, I suggest you get a pencil or pen and some paper and keep these by your side as you move through this basic lesson.

How the Method Works

Meridian tapping makes use of a natural human tendency that we all possess, that of using our hands to comfort ourselves. Although we don't usually realize it, every single day we are actually soothing ourselves, clearing our minds and making ourselves feel more comfortable by contacting natural Comfort Spots on our body, with our hands.

So that you can see what I mean, look at the photos and descriptions below and see if you recognize yourself or some other people you know:

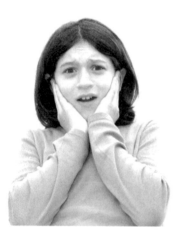

This girl brings her hands up to her temples and cradles her chin as she hears some upsetting news.

This child brings her hands up to cover her forehead at a time of distress.

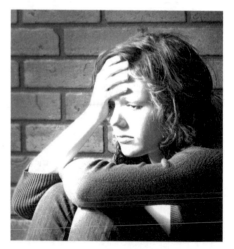

This man clasps his chin as he tries to figure out something.

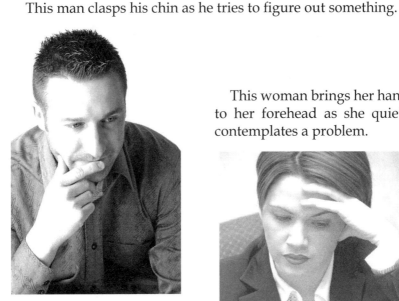

This woman brings her hands to her forehead as she quietly contemplates a problem.

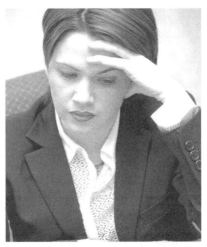

These are just some of the ways we contact comfort spots automatically and unconsciously. It is a universal human tendency to use our hands for support and comfort. Here you will learn how to use this tendency in a very special way — to *systematically* relieve stress. It will work for you because it's based on principles that your body *already knows*.

The meridian tapping method is a systematic way of using your own comfort spots by organizing them and putting them into a system. This is much more powerful than our usual haphazard way of using these spots. You will see how this works out.

As I have indicated, the meridian tapping comfort spots correspond to some of the acupuncture points that are used in traditional Chinese medicine. Meridian tapping is an extremely different process from acupuncture, however, because acupuncture uses needles and tapping uses a very gentle tapping, but the spots correspond to some of those ancient ones. Undoubtedly practitioners of ancient Chinese medicine were observing people over the centuries and noticed that they use their hands to comfort themselves in very specific ways.

The Comfort Spots You Will Use When Tapping

As you look at the pictures below, try to locate each tapping spot on your own body as shown, so that you can easily find it later on when you are doing the technique.

You are not to tap yet, and you don't have to try to remember the names of the spots because we're going to be going over them a number of times and you'll have plenty of opportunities to get used to them and learn them by heart.

The sequence of comfort spots begins with what we call the *Karate Chop Spot.* This is the part of the hand that Karate masters use when they strike a piece of wood and split it in half with one single blow.

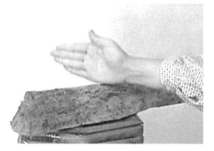

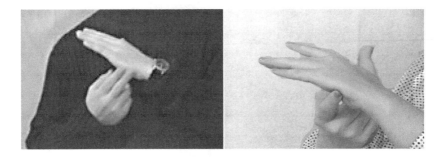

The *Karate Chop Spot* is located halfway between the base knuckle of the little finger and the wrist bone of either hand.

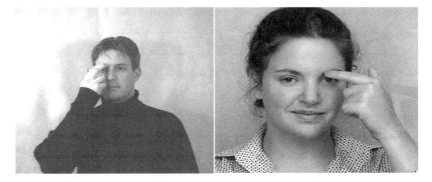

The next spot is at the inner corner of either eyebrow, right next to the bridge of your nose. It's called the *Inner Eyebrow* Spot.

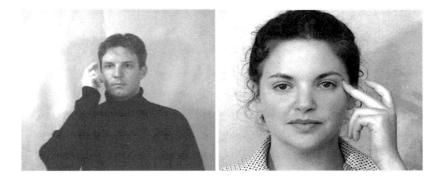

The next spot is at the outer corner of either eye, on the bone. It's called the *Outer-Eye Spot*.

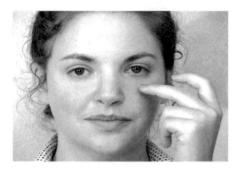

The next spot is right beneath either eye, in the middle, on the bone. It's called the *Under-Eye Spot.*

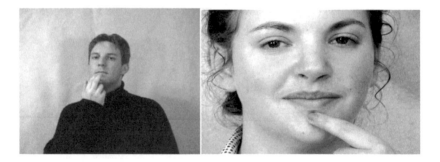

The next spot is directly beneath the nose and is called the *Under Nose Spot.*

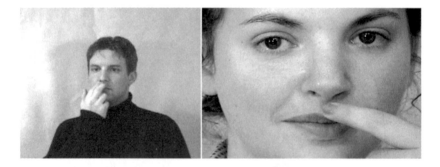

The next spot is directly under your mouth. It's called the *Under Mouth Spot.*

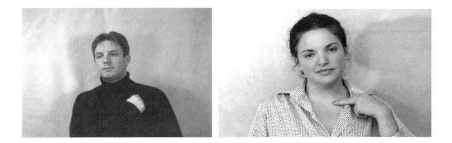

The next spot is the *Collarbone Spot*. You can find your collarbone by locating one of the two little upward pointing bones just beneath your throat, on either side of the body. Some people find them more easily than others. To make it easy to locate them, I suggest you make a fist (*as in left photo above*) and simply lightly thump this spot when you're doing meridian tapping. This way you'll cover quite a bit of territory with your fist so you'll be sure to stimulate the *Collarbone Spot*.

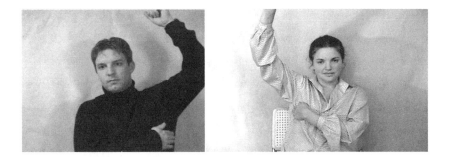

The next spot is called the *Under Arm Spot*. It is on either side of your body, roughly four inches under the armpit. Here you'll lightly thump your side with your hand in order to stimulate the area around the spot.

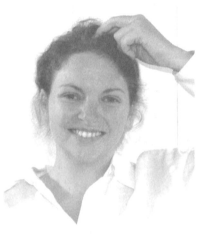

The final spot in this meridian tapping sequence is on the top of the head, towards the front. It is called the *Top Of Head* spot.

This is all there is to a single round of tapping.

THE TAPPING SEQUENCE

Step 1. Measure Your Stress Level Before Starting

You need some way of gauging your progress as you do meridian tapping in order to tell whether your stress level is actually coming down. This is something like taking your temperature when you're trying to find out if a fever is dropping, you will want to check on yourself.

For this you will use what is called an *Intensity Rating*. Here's how that works:

> You will gauge your intensity on a scale of 0 to 10, with 10 being as upset as you can imagine being about your issue, and 0 being completely laid back about it (i.e. it is no longer a problem).

HINT: When you take your Intensity Rating, do so casually and jot down the first number that pops into your mind. It is usually the most accurate.

Step 2. Select an Issue to Work on

For this first experience with tapping, you should select an issue from your own life to work on that meets the following criteria:

1. It should be a memory that troubles you and which you'd rather not have. This memory should have an Intensity Rating of at least "5" or more when you think about it *right at this moment*, but it should not be a *major issue* in your life. Because this may be your first experience with meridian tapping you don't want to apply it to too distressing an issue at first.

2. Next, select a *specific scene* that represents this issue. Sometimes issues are related to only one single scene. For example, say you had a ski accident on "Mount Airy" and you were afraid of skiing after that, and you'd like to use that particular issue to work on here. That would require you to think of only a single scene right now.

Many issues have more than one scene involved in them, however. Suppose that you are having difficulty with your boss at work. There will probably be a number of different scenes you can remember in which you have had run-ins with your boss. In this case, what you would do is select the most upsetting of those or the most vivid and recent one that really sticks in your mind.

Optional: Use the Distancing Technique if You Need to

An exception to the rule about selecting an upsetting scene is if the scene is *so* distressing to you that it would cause you a great deal of anxiety to think about it. Tapping is designed to be as painless a technique as possible. If thinking about your scene is extremely upsetting then you should use what is called the *Distancing Technique*. This is how that technique works:

If a specific memory is too upsetting, do NOT imagine a specific scene, but just use the words "that terrible thing happened" (or similar *general* wording).

Then, to take your Intensity Rating, do NOT create a visual scene in your imagination, just *say* the general words and GUESS what your rating would be.

Step 3. Select a Specific Scene

Select the most *vivid and distressing* example of your issue and recall it in as much detail as possible.

EXCEPTION: If you need to work with the Distancing Technique, use only *general* words, and do *not* imagine a specific scene in any detail.

Step 4. Create a Mental Movie

The next step is to create a mental movie in your mind in order to assign your issue an Intensity Rating. Your mental movie should have a beginning and an end, just like a scene in a movie.

You should make it as detailed as possible (unless of course you are using the *Distancing Technique*).

Step 5. Take An Initial Intensity Rating

Now that you have created your mental movie, run it through in your mind and give yourself an Intensity Rating according to how it feels to you *right this minute.* Write this rating down.

(NOTE: If you're doing the *Distancing Technique,* don't "get into it" and don't really think much about it. Use the general words you have chosen and just *guess* what your Intensity Rating *would* be if you were thinking about it. This works just as well).

Write down a number to indicate how you feel about your mental movie RIGHT NOW — at this minute. Select the first number that comes to mind.

Don't write down how you felt about your mental movie at *the time it happened,* or how you expect to feel about it in the future. You can't change the past or the future. You can only change the way you feel about your issue at this very moment. Use the first number that comes to mind. Your rating will be more accurate if you make it right off the top of your head.

Step 6. Give a Title to Your Movie

The next thing you are going to do is select a title or descriptive phrase that refers to your mental movie. This is just for your own use so you can focus on this movie while you're doing the techniques. It will be a reminder to you. Nobody else has to understand it, and it's certainly not going to be the title of an award-winning movie, so you don't have to worry about its artistic quality!

Now let's go back to that accident at Mount Airy. If this were your issue, you could just give it a simple title like *Accident at Mount Airy* to remind yourself of that scene. Or you might say, *My Sixth Birthday Party*, if that had been an upsetting time to you. Use a title that will remind you clearly of the event, that's all.

Write down this title.

Step 7. Create a Setup Phrase

Now you're going to create what is called a "Tapping Statement" or *Setup Phrase*. This statement starts with the words "Even though..." and is followed by a statement of your problem, which in turn is followed by a positive statement or affirmation, often one that tells how you would *like* to be or feel.

The formula goes like this:

1. Start your Tapping Statement with the words "Even though...."

2. Follow this by briefly stating your issue (e.g. "I'm worried about the exam").

3. Complete the sentence with a positive statement which is, in a sense, an affirmation. (e.g. "Even though I'm worried about the exam, I deeply and completely accept myself.")

Or,

("Even though I'm worried about the exam, I choose to be calm and confident".)

The first of these positive phrases ("I deeply and completely accept myself") is the default self-acceptance phrase used in the meridian tapping technique TFT and in traditional EFT, and can be very useful in many instances. It makes no difference whether you *believe* that you deeply and completely accept yourself or not, you just say it when the appropriate time comes. The reason for saying this phrase is that when we are caught in an intense emotion, we tend to blame ourselves for having it. This phrase gets us "off our own back" and allows us to forgive ourselves for the feelings we have — this way those feelings can be dealt with much more easily.

The second positive phrase ("I choose to be calm and confident.") is the default phrase used in the *Choices Tapping Method*. It tends to empower the user and to be very "believable". Either of these two phrases work excellently and you will choose which one you want to use for a particular situation. As you become more proficient at tapping you may make up positive phrases of your own to end your sentence. Tapping is a very flexible technique that lends itself well to individual variations.

This simple setup phrase will be used (while tapping on the *Karate Chop Spot*) to commence your tapping sequence.

Step 8. Create a Reminder Phrase

As you tap on the meridian spots in the sequence shown below, you will use what is called a Reminder Phrase to focus on your issue while you are tapping. The Reminder Phrase is just a shorthand description of your issue, such as "I'm worried about the exam", or "My fear of the exam" or just "Fear of exam," etc.

Step 9. Do the Preparation Exercise

Using your tapping phrase (which consists of the entire sentence you have created for your issue), locate *the Karate Chop Spot* (see Spot 1 on the chart below) and briskly tap this spot while you are repeating your tapping phrase (i.e. the entire sentence) THREE TIMES out loud. Then move on to Spot 2 on the chart.

Step 10. Do the Technique Proper

There are several ways to commence the tapping sequence and to end it. In the movie *The Tapping Solution* you will see it demonstrated by *commencing* with the Top of the Head spot. This is a very good way of proceeding and very effective. Below we will show you another way, one where you *end up* on the *Top of the Head* spot instead of starting with it (in both versions all the rest of the spots proceed in the same sequence). Ending on the top of the head is also an excellent way of doing meridian tapping. It is simply your preference as to which sequence you want to use, as both are equally effective. It is always good to have a choice.

> *NOTE: Both Roger Callahan and Gary Craig first used a long form of the tapping procedure which had the person tap on many of the fingers of one hand and use a sequence of eye movements accompanied by humming to complete the tapping sequence. Gary Craig now uses a short form of this sequence very similar to the form taught in this book (and in the movie* The Tapping Solution*). This short form is all you need to know at this point to get excellent results from the technique.*

So, now you are ready to start the technique. You will begin at the Inner Eyebrow (Spot 2 on the chart). Tap on this spot while you repeat OUT LOUD your Reminder Phrase (e.g. "Worry about the exam") while you tap lightly but vigorously on this spot for as many taps as it takes to complete saying your Reminder Phrase out loud.

THEN MOVE ON TO THE NEXT SPOT (Spot 3 on the Chart) and repeat the same process, saying your reminder phrase *once* at each spot while tapping at the same time.

Each time you move to a different spot in the sequence (see chart) repeat your Reminder Phrase once out loud.

When you tap on each spot in the sequence you will end up on the *Top of Head* spot *(in this form of* meridian tapping*).* It usually takes about 7 taps per spot to finish saying your Reminder Phrase, but the exact number is unimportant.

The sequence of tapping points is shown on the Chart. You can use either hand, and can tap on either side of the body. Follow your own preference.

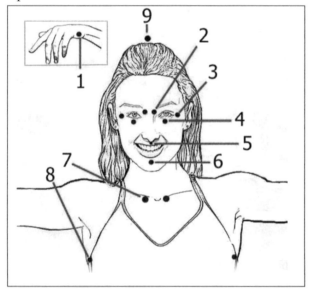

Spot 1: Karate Chop Spot
Spot 2: Inner corner of eyebrow
Spot 3: Outer corner of eye, on bone
Spot 4: Underneath the eye on the orbital bone, the bony structure beneath the eye (tap gently here, the tissue is delicate beneath the eyes).
Spot 5: Directly beneath the nose (above the mouth)
Step 6: Directly beneath the mouth
Spot 7: Collarbone spot. Make a fist and thump lightly on this spot, so that your fist covers the area just below one of the little points of the collarbone. Using your whole fist ensures that you are stimulating the entire area, it is therefore not necessary to be too precise with this location.
Spot 8: Underneath the arm at the side of the upper chest, about 4 inches below the armpit (exact position is not essential, see chart)
Spot 9: At the top of the head, near the front of the head. You may tap longer on this spot than the others if you wish.
This sequence completes one "round" of the treatment.

Important

As your Intensity Rating lowers over the course of a meridian tapping session, you should *modify your Tapping Statement accordingly.*

This is because your wording needs to reflect the changing reality of the situation — it will change as you tap. For example, if you were sad to begin with and now feel less sad, but still somewhat sad, say something like: "Even though I still feel *somewhat* sad, I deeply and completely accept myself". For the Reminder Phrase that you will use at each spot, now use the abbreviated phrasing, "I feel *somewhat* sad (or "a little sad") as you tap each spot. This way the sentence will reflect your changing feelings so you will not mistakenly recreate your original distressing emotion in its full intensity — you will not make yourself "go backwards".

When To End Your Tapping Session

Ideally, you should end the session when your Intensity Rating has come down to a "2" or below on all feelings involved, or at least as low as you can comfortably manage right now. If you find that you are not adequately reducing the intensity of your feelings, it is usually because you need to address another *Aspect* of your problem, something we will talk about in a moment. If you have reduced all the *Aspects* of your problem, you can expect considerable carry-over into the actual situation.

It is important to remember that meridian tapping is not simply a technique to make you "feel better"; it can actually change your *processing* of the situation. When it does so, its beneficial effects should remain. **Ordinarily there is at least an 80% carry over into the actual situation if you are using tapping on an issue that is currently active in your life.** If this doesn't happen, and you have checked out all the *Aspects* to this issue that you can think of, then further work with meridian tapping under the guidance of a trained professional may be needed to handle this situation.

It is the all important subject of *Aspects* that we will look at in the next chapter.

Chapter 7

Uncovering Hidden Aspects While Tapping

Sometimes a simple issue, such as a persistent fear or angry mood, has many angles or layers that need to be addressed. These multiple facets of a single problem are what we call *Aspects* in meridian tapping. Knowing about *Aspects* will make the whole method much more valuable and effective for you.

You can think of *Aspects* as pieces of a puzzle. The puzzle is your total issue — fear of dogs, for example. The *Aspects* are the different pieces that need to be put into place to clear the issue. Fear of dogs, for instance, may include dislike for the way they jump up on two legs, fear of being bitten, and a nauseated feeling that occurs when you smell dog food. Each of these *Aspects* should be tapped for separately.

Surprisingly often, though, there's only one piece of the puzzle that needs to be put in place, only one *Aspect*. When that's the case, you just tap down that one *Aspect* and the whole problem is usually gone permanently. It can happen even if that problem has been around all your life.

The following is an example of the kind of *single-Aspect* problem we see so often in meridian tapping.

An Elevator Fear Disappears After 30 Years

Some years ago I was doing a stress management seminar for a large Fortune 500 company on their premises and wanted to demonstrate how meridian tapping could be used. I asked if anyone in the group had an issue that they'd like to clear. I specifically asked for an issue that wasn't major, but that nevertheless bothered the person and that they'd really like to clear up.

One woman — let's call her "Jan" — raised her hand and said, "I've got an issue, but you probably can't do a thing about it because I've had it all my life."

The issue turned out to be a fear of elevators. "I've always been afraid of them, ever since I can remember." She said. "I walk up three flights of stairs every day to my workplace. I don't go into buildings where there are elevators if I can possibly avoid it. It's very inconvenient, but I'm afraid you can't do anything about it."

I said, "Let's try."

Jan came up in front of the group and I asked her what her Intensity Rating was when she just *thought* of getting into an elevator. She said it was a 9 out of a possible 10 (the highest rating for fear). So we tapped. We did a number of rounds of tapping as her intensity level lowered by increments. This took about 15 to 20 minutes. Finally her Intensity Rating had come down to a zero.

At that point she stared at me, amazed, and said, "I feel so ridiculous! I've had this fear all my life but I can't seem to conjure it up now. When I think of an elevator, I can't bring back the fear!" This is a very common response when tapping is working; the emotion that was present before just isn't accessible anymore. The memory of the incident or situation is now neutral. The charge has been taken off of it.

I said to Jan, "I'm glad it's down, but I'd like you to agree to a test. Down the hall is a bank of elevators. Would you be willing to walk down there and get into an elevator and have the whole group come with you?" There were 25 of us.

Jan said, "Fine."

So we filed out of the room and marched down the hall to the elevators. She rang the bell. As she did so I told her, "Your intensity may go up a little bit when you open the door, but don't get in unless you're still down to a *zero*."

The door opened and Jan was about to step in, but I could see a sort of frown on her face. Not a terrified look, but a hesitancy. I said, "Wait a minute. Are you still down to a zero?"

She thought about it and then said, "No, I'm about a three."

"Don't get in." I said. " Let's tap you down right here." And so we did, with the whole group watching and occasional passersby too.

Her level went down to a zero again. I said, "Okay, ring the bell." She obliged. The door opened and there was a big smile on her face this time as she looked into the elevator. I said, "Get in. We'll go with you."

Only about half of us would fit into that elevator, but we got in and rode along with Jan. She pressed the button herself. We went up to the sixth floor and came down again. She was smiling the whole time and walked out with a big grin on her face. Everyone clapped! It was a standing ovation.

The important thing about this story is what happened afterwards. I came back to conduct another seminar the following week, with a different group. There were some people in this second group who knew Jan. They told me what had happened with Jan since we tapped together.

She had gone home feeling much better about elevators, but her Intensity Rating did go up a bit a couple of times when she approached an elevator. Each time, she tapped herself down and after those first few times she didn't have any problem at all with elevators again. She was now using the elevator every day to get to her office. She was losing a little bit of healthy exercise, true, but she had gained the ability to go in tall buildings.

This was over ten years ago. Jan, whom I've kept in touch with, has never had that fear come back.

This is typical when you have *one single Aspect* to your issue and you clear it up with meridian tapping. It's gone.

There are a couple of interesting things about this story. The first thing is that Jan never remembered what had caused her fear of elevators in the first place. She knew it must have occurred before she was three years old, because that is when she first remembered being afraid of elevators, but she had no idea what caused it. But finding the cause wasn't necessary. The issue cleared up completely without it!

Sometimes people will remember the cause and sometimes they won't. We can get clearing either way. This is very encouraging and important to know.

The other thing to note is that even though the meridian tapping took very little time, this long-term fear cleared up permanently. So it isn't a question of *how long* the issue has been around, it's a question of *whether more than one Aspect is involved*. Apparently in Jan's case, there wasn't more than one. Hence a "miracle cure."

A Fear with Multiple *Aspects*

Of course many issues in our lives are not so simple.

Let me give you an example of an issue that had more than one *Aspect*. About a year ago, "Jason," an otherwise confident young man, came to me with a problem he had crossing streets. He would get very, very tense and tighten up at the curb, often hesitating a long time before crossing. Because of his anxiety, his judgment would suffer and he would be in actual danger crossing the street.

Jason is a very together kind of guy, a fine executive, but he had this one fear. The interesting thing is that he actually knew where it had come from, but he still couldn't do anything to get rid of it.

When he was about six years old, he had been hit by a car. The car came around a corner, running a red light and hit him, dragging him for about twenty feet and breaking two of his ribs. It was a serious accident and a shock. Ever since then, he had not been able to easily cross streets. He *could* cross them, but it was confusing and even a little dangerous for him because of his high anxiety level.

I asked Jason to think of the actual scene when he had been hit as a child and tell me what the most distressing thing about it was. He said was it was his sense of shock and bewilderment, coupled with a sense of utter helplessness. He was being pulled under that car and there was nothing he could do about it.

Those two intertwined feelings, bewilderment and helplessness, were the main two *Aspects* Jason remembered. He rated his feelings about both as a 10 on the intensity scale. So we worked on these *Aspects* first. "Even though I feel bewildered, I deeply and completely accept myself." "Even though I feel helpless," and so forth. He tapped both of these feelings down until his intensity was a zero.

Then I asked him to imagine the street-crossing scene again. Even though his bewilderment and helplessness were down to a zero, there was still something that didn't sit right. The memory was still a little bit anxiety-provoking. The Intensity Rating he now gave the scene was a 3.

So although we had come down on the *Aspects* of bewilderment and helplessness, the score for the issue as a whole was still hovering at a three. I asked him whether there was something else he remembered about the accident that bothered him.

He thought for a moment and said, "Yeah, my mom came running out of the house and up to the car, screaming, 'What did you do? What did you do?'" He said, "I had a terrible feeling of having done something awful but I didn't know what it was."

He thought about this again and said, "Actually, she was probably yelling at the driver, but I didn't know that. I had this sick feeling of having done something wrong."

I said, "When you think about that feeling that you had when she was yelling, what is your intensity level?

Jason replied, "That's a ten, too." So we tapped that down to a zero. Then I asked him to think about the scene again. He did and reported, "It's fine. I think I could cross a street without any problem now."

I said, "Would you like to try it?" There happened to be a busy street right in front of my office building.

We went downstairs and out onto the sidewalk. Jason watched the light and crossed the street. He had no problem; his judgment was excellent. He felt calm and said the anxiety was gone. It was. That's because we had traced that final *Aspect*. If we had only addressed the bewilderment and helplessness, we would have seen *some* improvement, but Jason still would have been somewhat nervous crossing streets. But because we had traced down that final important *Aspect*, we were able to gain a total clearing.

Keep this in mind when you do tapping.

Working with More Complex Issues

As you probably realize by now, it's important not to confuse your Intensity Rating for the issue as a whole with your Intensity Rating for one single *Aspect*. They're not the same thing.

Here's a basic formula to use in these circumstances:

If you have trouble reducing your Intensity Rating... Search for other *Aspects* and tap them down. Then, re-take your Intensity Rating for the Entire Issue. It should now be down to a zero or one.

This process works for most issues. But as you can imagine, some issues in life have a large number of powerful *Aspects*.

For example, suppose somebody has a history of childhood abuse. There will be many different incidents that contributed to this person's current problem and therefore many *Aspects* that need to be tapped down. Or think about traumatic war memories. Rarely are these single, isolated incidents, but multiple repeated traumas. Or a person might have had repeated illnesses or surgeries. These might make up a total issue of being afraid of hospitals. Each memory would be a separate *Aspect* of the problem, to be tapped down separately.

I suggest that if you have a serious issue that involves multiple traumas in your past, you seek professional help in working with this. Fortunately a number of therapists today are trained in using tapping along with their traditional methods of therapy. They can help you to tease out other *Aspects* through their questions and can provide knowledgeable support, which you will need.

Now we will consider an additional strategy that you can use when doing tapping that will make the method even more precise and in many instances more effective — the Choices Tapping Method. You will learn what it can do in the next chapter.

Chapter 8

It's Good to Have a Choice

In this chapter you will learn about an important form of tapping that can take you much further when you use it. It uses a special type of tapping statement known as a "Choice."

The addition of Choices statements in meridian tapping allows you to target a specific emotional problem and handle it in a more precise and comprehensive manner than is often possible using the traditional TFT and EFT default acceptance phrase ("I deeply and completely accept myself"). The Choices Method can be used in addition to, or in place of, that standard default phrase. Most meridian tapping practitioners nowadays make frequent use of both the standard default phrase and the Choices Method.

The Choices Method expands tapping's effectiveness in an exciting manner because it gains its power from a unique form of affirmation.

When we think of the word "affirmation" we often think of the kind of affirmation typically promoted in "positive thinking" books. That type of affirming calls for you to create a sentence that represents your desired state of reality and to state it *as if it were already so*. For instance, if you are having financial struggles, you might be told to repeat the affirmation, "I am wealthy… I am wealthy… I am wealthy…" The idea is that if you assert the desired state *as if* it were already existing, then forces both internal and external will set to work to make it so.

There is, in fact, some power and truth to this. However, the problem with that kind of affirmation is that very often a large part of your mind simply recognizes the statement as false. You know perfectly well that the statement does not represent the way things really are in your life. You can say, "I am wealthy" till you're blue in the face, but all it takes is one look around your rundown one-room apartment to see that you're *not* wealthy. It's obvious. So when you make this kind of as-if-it-were-true affirmation you often set up an internal contradiction. Part of you is "willing" the statement to be true, another part of you recognizes it as patently false. This can set up doubt and skepticism, which often defeats the affirmation process right at the starting gate.

Choices affirmations are powerful because they do not contradict your present view of reality. As a result they are more readily accepted by most people than are "standard" affirmations. Choices statements have a very special application in meridian tapping.

When using the Choices method, you make a statement about what you desire which begins with the phrase "I choose to..." instead of with a declarative phrase such as "I am..." "I have...," etc. Rather than saying, for example, "I *have* many wonderful friends" or "I *am* completely at ease in taxicabs," you might say, "I *choose to feel* a bond of friendship with many wonderful people," or, "I *choose to feel* calm and relaxed when riding in this cab."

We are always free to make *choices* in the here and now, so when we state things in an "I choose" format, we do not set up a disconnect with observed reality.

In a moment we'll look at some considerations that go into crafting powerful Choices statements, but first let's look at how to use Choices within the context of meridian tapping.

How to Use the Choices Method

When using the Choices method, we typically start our tapping statement the same way we do when using traditional EFT. That is, we say "Even though..." and then state our current problem. For example, "Even though I often feel angry and resentful walking into my childhood home..."

The *second half* of the statement is where the Choices method varies from traditional EFT and TFT. Here a specific, positive, Choice-oriented statement is substituted for the traditional self-acceptance affirmation ("I deeply and completely accept myself"). For example, we might say, "I choose to feel warm love and acceptance for my parents." This Choice statement is then used in all the subsequent reminder phrases.

So, the set-up phrase in this example would be, "Even though I often feel angry and resentful walking into my childhood home, I choose to feel warm love and acceptance for my parents."

This "Choice" is an expression of what you *truly desire* as an outcome for the problem situation. It is targeted at the specific problem rather than being a *general* affirmation, such as the traditional EFT self-acceptance phrases.

The procedure for doing the Tapping Choices technique involves doing three specialized rounds of tapping in sequence. The Intensity Rating (your measure of distress on a 0 to 10 point scale) is taken at the beginning and then again only after *all three rounds* are completed. Because the process involves three steps it is often called the Choices Trio.

Here's how you do it. You start with the Set-up, then move on to Choices Trio. Ready?

The Set-up Process:

1. Identify the negative thought, attitude, feeling, etc., that you want to be rid of. Take your Intensity Rating (level of intensity about this issue on a scale of 1 to 10).

2. Formulate a simple statement of the problem, for example, "I'm afraid of swimming in deep water."

3. Formulate a Choice statement that is an antidote to the problem statement. For example: "I choose to feel completely at ease swimming in deep water."

4. Combine the problem statement with the Choice to create a Choices Set-Up phrase: "Even though I'm afraid of swimming in deep water, I choose to feel completely at ease when swimming in deep water."

5. Tap the Karate Chop spot while repeating this Choices Set-Up phrase three times. Now move on to the Choices Trio.

The Choices Trio:

Round 1: Do *one* complete round of tapping using the problem statement *only* as your Reminder Phrase. For example, "I'm afraid of swimming in deep water" or "this fear of swimming" repeated at each tapping point.

Round 2: Follow immediately (*without* checking your Intensity Rating or repeating the Set-Up) with one complete round using the Choices statement *only* as your Reminder Phrase. For example, "I *choose* to feel completely at ease when swimming in deep water" repeated at each tapping point.

Round 3: Follow immediately (without checking your Intensity Rating or repeating tapping phrase) with *one* complete round of tapping in which you *alternate* the problem statement and Choices statement as follows:

> At the first tapping point (Inner Eyebrow) use the problem statement as a Reminder Phrase (e.g. "I am afraid of swimming in deep water").

> At the next tapping point (Outer Eye), use your *positive Choice* for the Reminder Phrase (e.g. "I choose to feel completely at ease when swimming in deep water").

> At the next tapping point (Under Eye), *again* use the *problem statement* for the Reminder Phrase… and so on. Continue this alternating of negative and positive for the entire round.

Now retake your Intensity Rating. If more work is needed, repeat the Trio (above) as many times as necessary. That's all there is to it!

There's one more thing you should know about the Choices Method however. It is very flexible and you can tailor it to your own needs. If you want to you can abbreviate the process so that you do only *two* rounds using your Reminder Phrases instead of three — the first round repeating only the negative reminder phrase (the problem) at each tapping spot, and the second round repeating only the positive Choices phrase at each tapping spot. Or to make it even easier for yourself, you could just repeat the entire set-up phrase (the whole sentence starting with 'Even though...") at each tapping spot. You will want to make it as easy and comfortable and natural for yourself as possible. It can be a powerful aid to tapping even when it is varied this way.

Creating Powerful and Effective Choices Statements

The *quality* of your Choices statement will go a long way toward determining how helpful the Choices Method will be for you.

Most people don't know how to identify what they really want but, ironically, they are almost always clear on what they *don't* want. When asked to make a positive Choice, most people will just choose to improve slightly upon their current "negative" state of affairs. One way they do this is to resort to comparisons. They will use such words as "better" or "more," in their Choices statements. For example: "I choose to feel *better*." "I choose to be *more* confident." "I choose to have *more* money in the bank," etc.

This type of statement doesn't work very well though because our subconscious, computer-like mind cannot interpret it with any precision. What does "better" mean? A tiny bit better? How much is "more"? A penny more? When this isn't spelled out precisely your Choice can't go to work efficiently and effectively. So...

The First Rule of Choices is *Be Specific*. When making a Choice, it's better to state what you want precisely and quantifiably. A relatively poor Choice for a student, for example, would be: "I choose to get better grades this semester." A much more effective Choice would be, "I choose to get a 3.8 grade point average this semester" (or whatever grades are desired). In the same way, instead of saying, "I choose to have more money in the bank," say, "I choose to earn $85,000 this year" (or whatever exact amount you desire).

Specific Choices are stronger because they are self-explanatory and concrete. They don't require comparisons to some other state and they don't create uncertainties as to degrees of improvement.

The Second Rule of Choices is to *Create a "Pulling" Choice.* Choices must "pull" in order to be effective. They must draw your attention, captivate your imagination and provide real motivation. A lifeless Choice is like a dull advertisement; you just skip over it and it has little impact. Think of a Choice as an ad made up *by* you and directed *to* you as the consumer. The person who must be sold is *you* — you've got to buy into it and truly *want* the result you are trying to bring about.

I recommend making the *language* of Choices as colorful, appealing and attention-getting as possible. Sometimes that means using a few short, strong words sparingly: "I choose to *blast* through my finals." Or, sometimes carefully selected *adjectives* can make the Choice really stand out: "I choose to be *delighted* by how relaxed, creative and inspired I feel when taking my finals." The aim is to draw yourself like a magnet toward the goal you seek. The repeating of your Choices phrase during the tapping process should give you pleasure, comfort, and inspiration so that you actually *want* to keep saying it over and over.

Some phrases that can be included in a Choice to make it "pull" are:

I choose to:
- let it be easy to…
- surprise myself by…
- find a creative way to…
- find it fun to…

Adding adjectives such as the following can give it more charge:
- comfortable
- satisfying
- delightful
- ingenious
- safe
- unexpected

The Third Rule of Choices is to *Go for the Best Possible Outcome.* The rule of thumb here is to be inwardly *truthful* in what you are choosing. You need to choose what you *really* want in your innermost desires, not what you think you *should* want or what others want *for* you. And your Choice should reflect the very best level you can imagine attaining.

It is not enough to choose to find a "new apartment," for example, because a "new apartment" might be a dingy, sixth story walk-up with poor heating — yet technically it might be "new" for you. A much more effective Choice would be to state exactly what you *really* want, such as "I choose to live in a quiet, sunny, delightful apartment with a great view."

When crafting your Choices statement, spend some time letting your imagination go wild creating a strong, specific and colorful image of what you really, really desire. That way, you will make a Choice that won't shortchange you and will bring far more satisfactory results.

The Fourth Rule of Choices is to *State Your Choice in the Positive.* Negative words or phrases should be avoided whenever possible when forming the Choice part of your tapping statement. However, negative words and phrases are used in the beginning (negative) part of the statement in order to neutralize their impact by tapping repeatedly on the negative. The reason for avoiding negatives in the Choices phrase is the literalness of the computer-mind which doesn't know what to do with negatives. It understands "mountain," for example, but doesn't comprehend, "*not* mountain." Negatives have no reality to the subconscious mind so the mind can't get a fix on them. Rather, the mind focuses on the word that *follows* a "no", "never", "non-" or "not". It's like telling yourself not to think about a purple giraffe. Your mind immediately conjures up a purple giraffe!

So we are always better off keeping it positive when framing any sort of suggestions (and Choices really are self-suggestions) to ourselves. A poor way to word a Choice would be, "I choose to not be afraid of riding in planes." A much better way to word it would be, "I choose to feel calm and confident when riding in planes."

The Fifth Rule of Choices is to *Do Not Make Choices for Others.* It is important, when crafting a Choices statement, not to try to change the behavior of other people. We have no jurisdiction over others, nor should we ever assume that the world would be a better place if we could control *their* choices. Everyone has freedom in his or her own life.

Thus, it's best to avoid Choices statements such as:

"I choose to have Mary love me."

"I choose to have the people at work think I'm the best."

"I choose to have Kenneth apologize.", etc.

There are many ways that the above Choices can be reworded so as to make them non-manipulative, ethical, and personally effective. For instance, in the first example, you could say instead, "I choose to *feel* that Mary loves me." In that way you are making a Choice about your own *reaction* to Mary, something that lies well within your jurisdiction. Such a Choice can be very effective by the way because it is apt to make you react very differently to Mary, and she in turn may begin to react differently to you.

Our Choices should generally be as beneficial as possible to others and to the world, without imposing *our* values on them. We must honor others' individuality and freedom of choice. Not only is this a more respectful way to Choose, but it is more effective, too, because it keeps the focus on the one thing we *can* change — our own life's experiences.

Now we will look at how tapping relates to Past, Present and Future.

Almost every issue has a root somewhere in early childhood... So many little events happen to kids that we as adults would think nothing of — but they are traumatic for children.*

Norman Shealy, M.D., Ph.D.
*Founder of the American Holistic
Medical Association
Founder of the Shealy Institute
for Pain Management*

Tapping can unlock childhood traumas which have been stored within us from our earliest days, allowing them to heal.

*Quote from Dr. Norman Shealy from the movie, *The Tapping Solution.*

Chapter 9

Meridian Tapping for Past, Present and Future

You might call meridian tapping a technique for all times and occasions. It can be applied to past issues to remove their emotional charge, to present issues to help you cope better with what is happening now, or to future issues to troubleshoot any upcoming challenges. Here is how to do this.

- **For past or long term ongoing issues** — meridian tapping, as we've already seen, can be used to address issues that originated in the past and are causing recurring problems in the present. We have looked at some illustrations of this already, and will look at many more as the book unfolds. Jason's anxiety with crossing streets, for example, stemmed from an incident in his childhood when he was hit by a car. If you have seen the movie *The Tapping Solution* you will remember the way that Jackie's experience of hearing her father beating her brothers behind closed doors still impacts her today, many years later, by instilling in her a terror of making slip-ups (not being "perfect"). Or how Jodi's father's preferential treatment of her sister (he would always hug that sister first upon greeting the children, and neglect Jodi) affects her present life and health. Both physical and emotional pain often have their basic roots in childhood.

- **For present situations** — meridian tapping can be used *right on the spot* when a stressful situation is occurring — a plane hitting a patch of turbulence, a difficult business meeting, an uncomfortable family gathering. Tapping can bring our stress level down in the here and now whenever the world is feeling unsafe or challenging. It can be an ever-ready help in times of trouble.

- **For future situations** — meridian tapping can be employed to deal with an upcoming event or circumstance that causes us worry or concern — and most anxieties are directed to the future. We call using tapping to troubleshoot situations that we anticipate to be challenging *Anticipatory Tapping*. Many people also use meridian tapping to attract and manifest new results in their lives, thus deliberately "sculpting" a better future for themselves. We will talk more about this later.

Now for a closer look at how meridian tapping relates to our past, present and future, and how we use it slightly differently for each of these situations.

Tapping for the Past

Although this may seem like an obvious point to many readers and certainly to anyone who works in the healing professions — it is worth stating clearly here. *Our lives are profoundly affected by the events and circumstances of our childhood and the ways we have invented to cope with these events.* Children are extremely vulnerable and highly sensitive — they pick up what is around them like an antenna and record far more of it than adults often realize. Many things that would not be traumatic or painful to adults are terrifying to children. When a young child suffers any form of trauma or abuse, s/he does not have an adult's mental and emotional capacity to process the resulting shock and pain or put the incident in perspective. Instead, the mind/body's energy system registers and "stores" the pain in a very direct way.

Think of the body's energy system as a river that is constantly flowing. When there are no blockages, the river flows freely. This feels good and leads to health and a feeling of buoyancy in life. But when a trauma or other negative event occurs, this creates a blockage, much like a boulder dropped into the river.

The boulder disrupts and diverts the flow of water. Once that boulder is in place, the river will flow around that blockage indefinitely. It will maintain an altered, disrupted pattern as long as that boulder remains in place. Which could be for a lifetime.

Similarly, when childhood pain, insult or injury causes a disruption in the energy system, this could permanently affect the flow of energy until this disruption is corrected. That disrupted, reshaped flow of energy almost always results in physical or emotional pain, or some kind of compromise to our overall sense of health, happiness and wellbeing. The disruption remains ongoing, it is always with us even though we may not be consciously aware of it much of the time.

Almost every emotional issue we face in adulthood has at least some, usually many, of its roots in early childhood. And yet, understanding these roots is often difficult and elusive — we feel pain or we behave in self-defeating ways and we don't know why. That's because our energy system is much more primitive than are the higher centers of the brain. The pain has been "stored" in our energy system since childhood, and when something in the present "re-awakens" it, it is felt again in all its fresh and primal fury. This is a process that occurs outside the scope of intellectual understanding.

Some of the stored pain from our past stems from *one-time* incidents in which we were traumatized, abused, humiliated, frightened or devalued. For example, we fall through the ice, we are bitten by a dog, or we witness our mother being beaten. These are the dropped boulders in our lives. But pain can also result from *long-term* repeated exposure to false, hurtful or negative messages about ourselves and the world that we "downloaded" before we knew any better. When we are young, we don't have our own world view — we are sponges that absorb all of our information and attitudes from those around us. We are essentially defenseless; we just take it all in.

If we are *repeatedly* ignored, shamed, or given fearful and limiting messages, this has a cumulative effect on our energy system. Think now of *handfuls of pebbles or sand* being thrown into the river, over and over, rather than boulders. Handfuls of these small obstructions don't change the course of the river immediately, as a boulder does, but they do build up and change its course over time.

If you are called "useless" once, it may not affect you in the long term unless the circumstances were traumatizing and left an indelible impression. If you are called "useless" a thousand times over the years, you can be sure this will create an emotional "sandbar" "or a "large dam of pebbles" that will alter your energy system in some fashion or form.

Most of the major emotional problems we experience in adulthood come down to issues of power or worth. We don't feel *capable* of achieving what we want or we don't feel *worthy* of achieving it. These feelings almost always originate in childhood.

So how do we resolve them? The problem with traditional means of treating childhood pain, such as using talk therapy alone, is that these rely solely on use of the mind, and the mind can take us only so far. Much of the real, deep pain of our lives was locked in place before we developed any kind of adult understanding, or it was installed during moments of shock when our logical reasoning powers were not functioning properly and we could not evaluate the situation properly.

Meridian tapping provides a mechanism not so much for *understanding* where our blockages came from but for *removing* the blockages directly. Remarkable insight, however, can spontaneously result from clearing an issue by tapping *after* the issue has been neutralized and its emotional charge removed. Tapping, in a sense, lets us wade out into the river and get rid of the boulder or the sandbar or the pebble dam, once and for all.

How do we apply tapping to issues rooted in our past? We have actually discussed this already in Chapter 7 on *Aspects*. If you have seen the movie *The Tapping Solution* you will have seen tapping being applied to many people at the Tapping Retreat who were suffering from childhood traumas.

A past issue may have only one single *Aspect*, in which case it will usually respond to tapping quickly and easily, sometimes in a single round. Or the issue may have multiple *Aspects*. In these cases we keep on tapping and uncovering the various *Aspects* until a clear sense of deep relief from the grip of the issue is achieved.

As I mentioned earlier, when dealing with serious emotional issues rooted in the past, it is often beneficial to seek professional help. A skilled meridian tapping practitioner can give you emotional support, encouragement to tap through the pain, and active guidance so that you can more thoroughly flush out all of the *Aspects* of your problem.

To sum up, any problem that is ongoing or recurrent in your life probably has its roots somewhere in your past.

Tapping in the Present

Frequently the stressful situation you need to deal with is not in the past but is happening *right now*. Though emotions from your past may be coming into play, the main threat, challenge, or pain is occurring right now. Some examples of stressful present situations might be: driving through sleet and snow, undergoing a medical procedure, sailing in turbulent waters, playing in the Big Game of the season, getting married, giving a speech to a large crowd, staying at the in-laws' house overnight, taking the bar exam, or starting a new job. I'm sure you can think of many more!

Tapping can be of enormous help in lowering your anxiety levels *right now* and allowing you to deal more effectively with a present challenge or even with a critical situation. Anxiety tends to feed off itself and produce more of the same. Sometimes we even become anxious about *being anxious* ("We have nothing to fear but fear itself," said American President Franklin D. Roosevelt to the people about the Great Depression of the 1930s). The more anxious we feel, the more removed we become from the situation at hand. We may get "stuck in our heads" and make poor decisions or deliver self-defeating performances. We may "choke" or tense up.

Tapping allows us to tame the extraneous, unproductive anxieties and become more focused in the present moment. The more centered we are right in this moment, the better we can handle whatever comes up. Challenging situations lose their threatening flavor and become more neutral.

When I talk to people about using tapping in the present,

the question I'm most often asked is, "How can I possibly use tapping at a funeral or a board meeting? It will be very noticeable and more than a little odd if I start tapping on myself in public." Yes, it is noticeable; that's why you will want to find a way to do it inconspicuously. One way to do this is to make an excuse to leave the room so you can be alone. There's almost always a way to get out of a room for a few minutes.

Another option is to tap inconspicuously on the karate chop spot on the side of your hand underneath a table or somewhere else where this will not be noticed, or to simply place your fingers lightly on each tapping spot without tapping at all (this works very well). Or you can do "mental tapping" by just *imagining* tapping the sequence of spots in your mind and repeating the phrases to yourself mentally.

In the future perhaps tapping will be so common that we won't need to seek out privacy, but in today's world you will still need to create a way to do this privately. Tap down the issue to a zero, or as low as you can get it in the time you have available. Then re-join the stressful environment and you will usually find that you'll handle it quite differently. Your change in mood, attitude or behavior will not only help you cope with the situation, it will often help to resolve the situation itself.

Tapping for Concerns About the Future

Much of the time, unfortunately, worries about the future are hampering our present. Just thinking about an anxiety-producing situation that we anticipate, our hands get clammy, our breathing becomes labored, our mood becomes dark solely *in anticipation* of what we perceive will be a stressful circumstance. In these cases, "Anticipatory Tapping" can be extremely useful. When we use Anticipatory Tapping, we're not trying to change the future, per se, but rather our present emotional state *regarding* the future. Interestingly, though, if we can change *that*, we often can influence the future as well, because we will enter the anticipated situation in a calmer and more focused state of mind. Fear can create a self-fulfilling prophecy, as can calmness and a sense of confidence.

One reason tapping works so well to counter "future fears" is that these fears are often irrational. We know they don't make sense but we feel them anyway. Because they're illogical to begin with, they don't respond well to reason. A more direct approach, such as that offered by meridian tapping, is thus more effective.

To do anticipatory tapping, simply acknowledge the future-worry that's bothering you, incorporate it into a tapping statement, and tap for it. This might require slight wording changes in the standard tapping phrasing. Just use common sense when doing this. Instead of using phrases such as "Even though I have this fear of mice," or "Even though I have this pain in my neck," you might say something like, "Even though I'm nervous about that interview next Tuesday," or "Even though I'm afraid of what the doctor's going to say."

In these cases, the reminder phrase you would repeat at each tapping point would be, "I'm nervous about that interview next Tuesday," or, "I'm afraid of what the doctor's going to say."

Can tapping be used to change the future itself? We will look briefly at that question later in this book, but for now let me say that I have received many promising testimonials from people who have used tapping as a positive tool to attract better finances, improved relationships, career changes and other beneficial results that have altered their futures profoundly. These folks are convinced that tapping was the key that brought about the change they were looking for. If you're open to the idea, why not try it? You might be the next person to report a remarkable and inexplicable result.

You have now learned the basics of meridian tapping and some simple variations that can expand its use remarkably. You literally have the power at your fingertips to begin applying this exciting technique to countless issues in your life.

Over the next few chapters we will be looking at some common uses of tapping — for pain, for fears and phobias, for weight loss, for performance issues, and for others — and sharing some inspiring true-life stories as we do so. Always keep in mind, though, that there are many, many more potential uses of meridian tapping than can possibly be covered in a single book. Fortunately, there are many resources that will help you in this, such as the website www.TheTappingSolution.com, my web site, www.TappingCentral.com and Gary Craig's, www. EmoFree.com, among others. They provide information that can greatly extend the scope of what you have learned thus far and take your practice of meridian tapping to a whole new level.

You have started an exciting journey that will be limited only by your imagination and willingness to try it on everything!

Now we will look at some of the specific ways tapping is currently being used by people in many parts of the world.

Part 3

Using Meridian Tapping in Your Life

If you could live your life over what would you wish hadn't happened? What would you remove?*

Brad Yates
Peak Performance Coach
Meridian Tapping Expert

These are the sorts of experiences that tapping heals as it acts to cleanse our energy systems.

*Quote from Brad Yates from the movie, *The Tapping Solution.*

Chapter 10

Try Tapping for Fears and Phobias

Do you remember the story about Mary, whose severe water phobia was eliminated in a single treatment of TFT, the technique that fathered meridian tapping? TFT was developed specifically to treat phobias so, not surprisingly, Meridian tapping is supremely well-suited to treating these types of emotional disorders. Clearing up fears and phobias, in fact, is the number one use for tapping among professional practitioners.

When a person experiences shock, trauma or intense fear — whether due to "real" or imagined circumstances — it can leave a deep, negative imprint on the body's energy system. This energy disruption is often highly "charged" and can be stubbornly self-sustaining and resistant to change, at least when addressed by conventional methods. Irrational fears may stay with a person for years, decades, or an entire lifetime, locked in the mind/body system essentially undiminished. The disrupted energy continues to flow along its altered "grooves," much like a river diverted by a huge boulder.

The idea that phobias and fears are even more deeply embedded in the energy system than in the conscious mind is evidenced by the fact that these fears are often recognized as "irrational" by the person who harbors them. These fears often show up to hamper us in situations where they make no sense and serve no logical purpose whatsoever. A swimmer with a shark phobia, for example, can become terrified in fresh water, where no sharks could possibly survive. A tourist with a fear of heights can go into a panic even when a thick wall of safety glass protects them from any possible fall. A hiker can break into cold sweats over the sight of a six-inch garter snake in the distance, known to be harmless.

The mind knows the fear is pointless, the body doesn't. This is because the fear is embedded in the energy system.

Why Tapping Works to Reduce Fear

Tapping is successful with fears because it does not just use a mental or rational approach, but goes directly to the source of the emotional charge — the disrupted energy signals running through the mind/body system. Because it targets the body's energy system *directly*, it can very often clear up fears and phobias with unprecedented ease and speed.

A vast number of clinical records and self-reports from around the world attest to this technique's remarkable ability to eliminate longstanding phobias, often (but of course not always) in as little as a single session. Tapping has proven effective in handling disabling fears of:

- medical or dental visits
- water
- elevators
- needles
- flying
- riding in automobiles
- tunnels
- public speaking
- death
- physical pain
- heights
- enclosed spaces
- creatures such as snakes, mice, spiders, cats and frogs
- and *many* other objects or situations

Of course, the degree of success that tapping achieves with any fear or phobia depends greatly on the individual experiencing it and the depth and severity of the problem. Surprisingly often the phobia is eliminated entirely when tapping is applied the first time. These immediate changes are what Gary Craig refers to as "One-Minute Wonders." At other times the fear may initially be sharply reduced, but persistent work over time using tapping is still needed. For deep, extreme and intransigent cases, the creativity and insight of a trained tapping therapist is needed if the person is going to have a real chance of a reversal or abatement.

Here are some incidents from real life that fit some of the above descriptions.

The Surprising "One-Minute Wonders"

Countless extraordinarily rapid elimination of fears and phobias have been reported by those who have used tapping. Web sites such as my own (www.TappingCentral.com) and Gary Craig's (www.EmoFree.com) list hundreds of these reports. Here are just a few.

Clearing An Irrational Fear of An Unusual Sort

Karen Ledger, a nurse and experienced meridian tapping practitioner, reports a ten-minute, apparently permanent, elimination of an intense and debilitating phobia of — strange as it may sound — TV screens! For fifteen years a new client of hers had been experiencing weakness, nausea and headaches whenever he found himself in the presence of TV screens and computer monitors. This was a particularly embarrassing problem because he was a scientist who worked in a setting replete with computer monitors. He had to purchase special equipment for himself and ask his colleagues to shut off their monitors whenever he was in their offices — a great inconvenience to all concerned. He attributed this physical/mental reaction to a change in his physiological makeup caused by his radiation treatment, fifteen years earlier, for Hodgkins Disease.

At the start of the tapping session, the patient's fear level was about a 7 (there was a 27-inch television screen in the room). Neither he nor Karen had a clue as to the reason for his irrational reaction.

But, during the first round of tapping, he had a spontaneous memory of a computer monitor that had been used to direct the course of radiation during his cancer treatments fifteen years earlier. His fear level dropped to a 3 at this point. After the second round, he reported no fear at all and asked Karen to turn on the TV, remarking on the screen's great resolution.

Ten minutes, from 7 to 0.

Three months later, this patient wrote back to her, thanking her and reporting that his fear had not returned, but his normal life had.

Pre-Operative Patient Benefits from Tapping

Mara Protas, an expert meridian tapping Practitioner who is a registered nurse, works in a hospital setting and frequently uses tapping on both patients and fellow staff members. Because her co-workers knew of her work with irrational fears, she was recently summoned to the room of a troubled pre-operative patient. When Mara arrived, she found the patient distraught and terrified. She was nearly hysterical about her upcoming surgery. Mara immediately asked the woman if she would like to try "a simple technique to help you with your fear — it involves light tapping on your face and upper body."

The woman readily agreed and the set-up phrase they used went as follows: *"Even though I'm terrified of surgery, I deeply and completely accept myself."*

In the middle of the second round of tapping the patient stopped abruptly and exclaimed, "Oh! It's gone!" Although they completed that round of tapping (it's always best to finish a round), the patient's panic had already completely subsided. She consented to surgery without a problem and the operation went smoothly.

Handling an Immobilizing Cat Phobia

André Fillon, not a trained practitioner but a "lay" user of tapping, has described the remarkable experience of quickly and effectively curing a powerful phobia in a guest at his home.

A dinner invitee had brought along a date whom André had never met before. André, the host, was pouring wine for his newly-arrived guests when he heard a ghastly scream and the slamming of a door. He ran outside to see what the problem was and found his embarrassed houseguest trembling on the back porch steps. The guest asked him to please get his coat from indoors, as he could not stay. He explained that a cat was the cause of the problem. The guest had such an intense fear of cats, he couldn't even be in the same *house* with one. In fact he could not so much as look at a cat on television without fleeing the room.

The host tried to talk to his guest about it and noticed that even talking about cats was making the man feel panicky. André then offered to try tapping with him. He promised this would be a gentle, non-confrontational experience and that if it didn't work, there would be no harm done. André would simply get the man's coat and send him on his way. The guest agreed.

André did a round of tapping with the guest, after which the intensity of his fear dropped from about a 9 to a 4. After a second round, the fear was almost completely absent — down to a 1 — and so André asked the man if he would be willing to walk to one of the windows and look in at the cat. The man did so and to his utter surprise he didn't feel anxious.

André then asked the guest if he would be willing to "touch" the cat through the glass and the guest agreed. When the cat came to the window the guest put his hand on the glass and the cat "sniffed" at it. At this point, the guest's anxiety went up slightly (to a 2) and André helped him tap it down to a 0.

The next step was for the guest to try entering the house again, with the doors kept wide open, of course, and a free invitation to leave whenever he felt uncomfortable. Once inside the house, the houseguest's fear went back up to a 3 or 4, but the host tapped him through the sequence again and soon he and the cat were making eye contact and the guest was wondering why he was ever afraid of cats. Before long he was stroking the cat's belly as the cat rolled over and purred.

By the time coffee rolled around, one cat was snuggled up to the guest's side while another slept on the chair behind his head. A closet "cat person" had been revealed! The amazing end to this story was that a couple of weeks later, the guest phoned André and asked him to go with him to the animal shelter to get a cat of his own. The man now has three cats that all sleep on his bed with him every night.

Not bad for a fifteen-minute time investment.

Some Cases Take More Time and Ingenuity

Not all cases are "One-Minute Wonders." In fact, a great many phobias and fears require longer, more complex processes or multiple sessions of tapping.

When There Are Many Aspects To A Single Problem

Not only are some fears more deeply entrenched than others, but many fears have numerous *Aspects*. This means that multiple memories, emotions and psychological considerations are driving the fear, each of which must be tapped for individually. Fear of flying, for example, might contain several, or all, of these common *Aspects*:

- Fear of being in an enclosed cabin
- Fear of not being in control during the flight
- Fear of the plane crashing
- Fear of heights
- Fear of being hijacked, etc.

If many different *Aspects* of a fear are operating but the person taps on only one of these, then the results will probably be incomplete.

When There Are Hidden Advantages to Maintaining a Problem

Another common problem when treating fears is the fact that we sometimes reap a host of "side benefits" by *maintaining* a fear, rather than curing it. Agoraphobia can be a good example of this. An agoraphobic person typically experiences seriously limited mobility in the community. This person then becomes accustomed to staying indoors, dodging social expectations, having other people come to him/her, etc.

These habits can become entrenched and eventually be even rewarding in some respects. Removing the fear could cause a crisis in this person's life in that his/her lifestyle might need sudden major adjustments. S/he might now feel required to meet a host of "normal" obligations, such as registering a car, going on job interviews, accepting social invitations, etc.

So sometimes there is a greater psychological pay-off in *honoring* the fear than defeating it. More often than not, however, the person to whom this happens is not fully aware of this side of the equation. However, the greater these hidden benefits, as a general rule, the less quickly a phobia will typically respond to meridian tapping.

Using Tapping for a "Crazy" Fear of Clowns

An example of a meridian tapping case that took longer than a "One-Minute Wonder," but was nevertheless successful, is reported by Jo-Anne Eadie, an EFT Trainer. During one of her workshops Jo-Anne encountered a person with such a serious fear of clowns that she could not even say or write the word "Clown", but could only refer to them with the letter C. A friend had to explain her problem to Jo-Anne.

The phobia had started when the woman was 5 years old and her father had put on a movie called "It," based on a Stephen King novel and featuring a bloodthirsty and disturbing clown. Her father immediately shut off the movie but it was too late. On a scale of 1-10, this woman described her C-fears as a 100-plus. The following quote from Gary Craig's website, www.EmoFree.

com (with minor punctuation, wording and emphasis changes), describes some of Jo-Anne's work with this individual:

   We began with "Even though I am terrified of clowns, I deeply love and accept myself," with small reminders of all the different things about clowns that she doesn't like. Her intensity was now at a 9½.

   "Even though my father didn't mean to scare me with the movie…"

   "Even though my mother tried to reassure me…"

   "Even though I thought about it all day…"

   "Even though I had nightmares that wouldn't go away…"

   "Even though I think they will kill me…" She is down to nine.

   "Even though other people think that C's are funny, I know they are going to get me…"

   "Even though I feel this fear in my solar plexus and my heart…"

   "Even though I get panic attacks if I am too close to a C…"

   "Even though people make fun of me and think this is all silly to be scared of C…"

   "Even though my friends in college played that cruel joke on me…" She is down to an eight.

   "Even though I have to be on guard so the C's and mimes won't trick me…"

   "Even though I didn't believe my mom and dad when they told me the clowns won't hurt me…"

   "Even though I can't say the word clown…"

   "Even though I hate clowns, I choose to love clowns." Reminder phrase is "I hate clowns, I love clowns, I hate clowns, I love clowns." Three rounds of flipping back and forth and she is now *saying* the word clowns on the "I hate clowns" but is silent on the "I love clowns" and lets me say it for her. She is down to a seven.

"Even though I don't want to let this go..."

"Even though I don't want to let this go, because it is my safety and protection against clowns..."

"Even though I am an adult now and the little girl doesn't need the protection anymore..."

While tapping the collarbone point she gripped the chair and started to have a panic attack. Tapping on her made no difference. I put my hands on her hands and asked her to tell me one thing in the room that she could see, one thing in the room that she could hear, one thing in the room that she could smell. Could she feel the chair beneath her? Could she feel her feet in her shoes on the floor? Then we went through the tapping sequence again and halfway through she was back in her body, calm and ready to continue. We were only coming down slowly by ones but it was the best she had ever felt about clowns and she could now say the word easily.

We took a short break and when we returned, she very much wanted to continue. We stayed on "Even though I don't want to let this go, because it is my safety and protection against clowns..."

"Even though I don't want to give up my safety and protection, I choose to let it go." We used the small reminder phrase, "I don't want to let this go, I choose to let this go," until I saw a sigh. She was down to a six.

I was racking my brain trying to think of something that would ALLOW her to let it all go. Laughter is always a wonderful release but I wanted to be careful not to make fun of her as so many others had done. "Even though I might meet and start dating a man and fall in love with him and marry him and it turns out he is a clown and a mime, I deeply love and accept myself and my clown husband."

She kept tapping but couldn't say the words because she was laughing so hard and saying that she would dump him in a minute if he was a clown.

Magically, she was a zero... Total time: 35 minutes

Progressing very slowly does not mean that tapping is not working.

Tapping for a Long-Term Phobia of Snakes

On my DVD entitled *EFT in Action for a Snake Phobia* I demonstrate a detailed, real-life session with a woman, Evelyn, who had an intense fear of snakes. As with the houseguest above who could not look at cats on the screen, she could not even watch snakes on TV. This fear of snakes turned out to have numerous *Aspects*, rooted in disturbing memories and experiences from different times in her life. To thoroughly clear her phobia, we needed to address each of these *Aspects* in turn.

Aspect **#1** turned out to be a memory of herself as a 5 or 6 year old mistakenly reaching for a coiled-up snake she had thought was a rock. When she saw it was actually a live snake and it crawled off between her feet, this gave her an intense jolt as she withdrew in *startled fright*.

Evelyn tapped the horror associated with this memory down to a zero. Then we went on to identify the next *Aspect* of her fear of snakes.

Aspect **#2** was the horror and *nauseated feeling* she had experienced in childhood when she saw a snake that had recently eaten a small animal. The lump in its throat was physically unpleasant to recall and made her feel intensely sick to her stomach. Evelyn tapped the nauseated feeling down to zero, then we continued.

Aspect **#3** involved memories of Evelyn's mother shooting snakes in her childhood swimming hole to protect her and the other children. The way a snake would writhe and flip over, revealing its underbelly, was very *creepy* to Evelyn — like watching a horror movie — and it still disturbed her to think about it. Two rounds of EFT and the horror vanished from this memory.

The most intense of the *Aspects, Aspect #4,* involved an incident that occurred when her 17-month-old daughter was just learning to walk. Unbeknownst to the toddler, but clearly known to her mother who watched from a distance of about 50 feet, the child was approaching a large and deadly snake while trying to walk to mom. Evelyn could do nothing to protect her child and dared not call out to her because that might make the little girl move suddenly and startle the snake which could then strike her.

So Evelyn watched in silent despair as her little daughter stepped nonchalantly over the snake and continued on her way, unharmed as it turned out. Evelyn described her reaction when she thought about this incident as a feeling of being "sick unto death." Several rounds of tapping were needed before her intense reaction to this near disaster faded. But it finally did. The expression on Evelyn's face was one of incredible relief when she tapped on the fact that she now knows that her daughter "survived." She could suddenly feel this on a very deep level, never accessible to her before.

As you can see, each *Aspect* of Evelyn's fear of snakes stemmed from a different memory and had its own signature emotions — startled fright, nausea, horror-like revulsion, and intense fear and guilt at being unable to save her child. For each *Aspect* we did separate rounds of tapping. Each time we started by discussing the particular "flavor" of that fear and assessing her current distress level regarding this particular *Aspect* (usually that was very high to start with). We then came up with appropriate set-up statements, such as "Even though I almost picked up that snake...," "Even though that memory makes me feel sick...," or "Even though that was a creepy memory...," usually followed by the statement, "I deeply and completely accept myself."

After going through the initial tapping sequence for each *Aspect*, we would then re-assess her fear level, which was almost always much lower than at the start. We'd then go through a *clearing process*, repeating the steps to remove the residual trauma, using lines such as, "Even though there is still a little creepiness left…"

When we got to the memory of her baby daughter, several rounds of clearing were needed to remove this complex and highly charged *Aspect* of her snake phobia. We made sure to include the concept of forgiveness for herself, as Evelyn clearly still felt irrational guilt about the incident. We also chose to include some positive statements such as, "Even though I felt sick unto death (about my daughter almost stepping on the snake), I choose to remember how *perfectly* [my daughter] survived."

Our 53-minute in-office session concluded with Evelyn first looking at, then holding in her lap, a very realistic rubber replica of a snake. She was able to do this with no pressure from me, and even agreed to go to a nearby pet store to see a real live snake. In the DVD you see Evelyn walking up to within four feet of a six-foot boa constrictor which is being held *outside of its cage*, by its handler. Evelyn observes the snake with a peaceful, interested expression on her face and says simply, "Why, she's pretty, isn't she?"

Six weeks later the film shows Evelyn at her office talking about how she has recently watched a tape I had lent her about the Amazon rain forest, which contained footage of writhing snakes. Not only had she been able to watch it, but she actually found herself *interested* in the subject matter and rewound the tape to watch it a few more times. Her fear had been blocking a natural curiosity.

When I followed up on this single treatment session by phoning Evelyn five years later, she told me that her fear is still completely absent even though she has returned to live in the mountain country of her childhood where snakes abound. She is intelligently cautious of the snakes, but has no irrational fear of them at all.

The value of involving a trained tapping practitioner in more difficult and complex cases cannot be overstated. Although tapping was developed to be a self-administered technique and often suffices as just this, it is frequently the insight, experience and creativity of a trained practitioner that takes the process to its most effective level. Tapping is like any skill — the more one does it, the better one gets at it. Sometimes only an experienced practitioner can unlock the power of this method in a given situation, especially when the emotions are powerful and complex. An additional example from my own practice comes to mind in which deep fears born of wartime trauma were reignited by a present-day event. It was only the confidence and insight I had acquired through years of psychotherapy practice that allowed me to intervene effectively with tapping.

Using Tapping for a Macho War Veteran

Tommy was a friendly and engaging, but tough-as-nails, Vietnam vet who weighed about 300 pounds, most of which was pure muscle. He was a self-appointed defender of the weak who always projected a macho image of strength and invulnerability. I knew Tommy because he had done work around my house for years. Even when beset by tragedies and challenges that would reduce most of us to quivering mounds of Jell-O, Tommy remained cheerful and "invincible."

So I knew it was trouble when he called me one morning, telling me that he was leaving town forever. He just had to "get out" and never come back. There was tremendous urgency in his tone as he poured forth a nonstop barrage of words.

I learned that during a winter snowstorm the night before, a car had skidded off the road and smashed headlong into a tree in his yard. Tommy had managed to pry open the car door and lift the driver out, but the man had died in Tommy's arms, just as some of his war buddies had done years before. Now Tommy was "seeing" his whole backyard aflame with bombs bursting just as they had on the battlefields. "I don't know what's happening," he kept repeating, "but I've gotta get out of here!"

I knew Tommy had called because he wanted my help, otherwise he would have simply skipped town as he was threatening to do. But I also knew that his self-image could seriously get in the way of any treatment. He would not/could not allow himself to be perceived as emotionally vulnerable.

I told him, in a voice that left no room for argument, "Tommy, you get over here, NOW! We can fix this." When he entered my home I saw this huge man trembling noticeably, his face ashen. There was no time to "sell" him on tapping or to give him a primer. All I said was, "I'm going to use a new method that can take away the kind of experiences you're having. It's being used with Vietnam veterans who have the same problems you do now, with a lot of success."

I wanted Tommy to believe that the technique would work and I didn't have the luxury of caution. I needed all the help I could get. Confidence on my part would be a great asset, as would the idea that other Vietnam vets had benefited from the method.

My strong sense was that Tommy would not permit himself to break down and express the real emotions that were underlying his intense fear. So I did not want to use an approach that might force him to relive last night's experiences or his war experiences. I knew that if we did, he'd be out the door in a flash.

So I chose to use the Distancing Technique. That is, I instructed him not even to THINK about the accident but merely to "guess" what his distress rating would be IF he were to think about these things.

Although he reported a "10-plus" on a 1-10 scale, he did manage to repeat, "Even though this man was killed on my property... I deeply and completely accept myself," and did a round of tapping on that. I purposely did not have Tommy describe his own emotional reaction to the event, but helped him construct a reminder phrase that reflected the facts alone.

After tapping a complete round this way, he was obviously experiencing some relief. His breathing was easier, his eyes more focused, and he described himself as "a little better." After tapping another round, Tommy felt better yet. Then, on an intuition, I suggested that we go directly to the memories of the war. I asked him if he had seen men die like this in the war. He told me that he had.

I then asked him to say, "Even though they died in my arms in the war...," reminding him not to *imagine* the war experiences, but only to *say* them. He did as I suggested.

In all, Tommy did about eight to ten rounds of tapping. I watched in amazement as his distress level came down, in just 12 minutes, to a zero. He had stopped trembling, looked like a new man, and could only keep repeating, "This stuff is something else! This stuff is SOMETHING ELSE!"

Tommy's tapping treatment was remarkably successful. He was able to go back to work that day with no difficulty, and did not "flee the state." I have been keeping close tabs on him for several years now and his flashback has never occurred again. Nor has the fatal accident on his property bothered him.

Here my training and experience as a psychotherapist allowed me to help in a way that a non-professional probably would have had considerable difficulty doing.

The Unexpected Side Benefits of Using Tapping

One of the hidden benefits of using tapping to clear up a fear or phobia is that related problems often clear up spontaneously, granting the individual a new sense of emotional freedom. Fear is a form of intense stress and as such it takes its toll on our minds and bodies in ways we are often unaware of. This fact is demonstrated in a story reported by Gary Craig.

During one of his EFT trainings, Gary was working with a participant named Nate, who was tapping on an old memory in which he had slipped on some ice and nearly fallen into the Grand Canyon. Once this issue was "put to bed," (i.e. resolved) he recalled another heights-related incident. (As Gary points out, this kind of "daisy chain" reaction often happens during tapping, where one memory leads to another and another, taking the participant on an unexpected journey of healing.)

The new memory involved an incident with a helicopter. Whereas the slipping memory had been resolved fairly quickly and easily, the helicopter event was a different matter. As soon as Nate began to work on this incident, he began perspiring visibly. As this was near the end of the training event, Gary offered to finish working with him in private.

Nate's physical symptoms — sweating and discomfort — continued as he described his work, years earlier, as an army psychologist. One day his fellow Delta Force teammates harassed him into parachuting out of a helicopter. Nate forced himself to jump in order to appease his buddies, but his body completely rejected the idea. He was in terror until his chute opened.

Gary helped Nate tap on the various *Aspects* of this memory until he stopped sweating, and finally he felt fine.

Two days later, when Gary asked Nate how he was doing, he reported some remarkable changes. Not only was he fine with the helicopter incident but his eyesight had noticeably improved and his blood pressure was measurably lower. Normally it fell within the range of 130/80 to 140/90, but now it was showing up as 106/"70-something." Nate had not tapped at all about health issues; this was a spontaneous change.

A few weeks later, Nate told Gary that his eyesight had remained improved and that he expected to get off his blood pressure medication soon. He also reported feeling more "aligned" and present. His preoccupation with money issues related to his eventual retirement had subsided and his psychotherapy practice had picked up, with new referrals coming "out of the woodwork."

Can it be proven that all of these benefits stemmed from tapping? Not exactly, but there is no doubt that fear constricts us on many levels. When we clear up fears and phobias, it seems self-evident that our lives are going to accelerate and improve in ways both obvious and hidden. Some of those effects can be considered direct results of tapping, others are indirect benefits.

In the next chapter we'll look at the benefits of tapping in an entirely different area. Its ability to improve personal performance can be dramatic.

Tapping "Choices" for Fears and Phobias

Even though I feel anxious *(scared, terrified etc.)*...
...I choose to be calm and confident.
...I choose to feel safe.
...I choose to handle this problem with surprising ease.
...I choose to remember good feelings I had today.

If a client comes to me and says, "On a scale of one to ten, my life is a three", my next question is, "Why so high?

They say, "What do you mean?"

And I say, "Well, why isn't it a two or a three?"

...and they go, "Well, yes, I guess it's not a one... well, my son's really a great kid, and I'm having a good time with him, and my mother's been supporting me through the divorce..."

And I go, "Great, so what would it take to move it to a four for you?"*

Jack Canfield
Co-author "Chicken Soup for the Soul"
Best-Selling Series Featured in
"The Secret"

Tapping can expand your life, moving it ever further in a positive direction.

*Quote from Jack Canfield from the movie, _The Tapping Solution_.

Chapter 11

Try Tapping to Enhance Performance

Meridian tapping is a brilliant tool for clearing fears and phobias, but its usefulness goes well beyond counteracting negative emotions. Tapping can be used to produce positive emotions and behavior just as easily as it can clear away negative feelings. The result is that it is now finding its way into classrooms and board rooms, onto stages and playing fields, as athletes, artists and a wide range of others who strive to excel in one area or another are discovering its remarkable power to remove internal obstacles that get in the way of high-level performance.

Practice, knowledge and talent are still needed for the highest level of achievement, of course. Tapping won't teach you how to play a Bach fugue or hit a fastball. But it may help you remove the negative beliefs that are telling you you're incapable of hitting a fastball. Or it may help you maintain mental presence and focus to such a degree that the fastball seems to "slow down," permitting you to hit it with exceptional ease.

As you will recall, in Chapter 1, baseball star Pat Ahearne reported how his game improved dramatically when he learned tapping, a tribute to the remarkable effects this method can have on improving the performance of even a professional athlete. His experiences in using tapping to remove personal blocks to top performance are now being duplicated by many others.

Many psychologists, coaches and others who help people enhance their performance have, in fact, come to believe that for every talented star performer there are thousands of equally talented individuals who never make it. These people remain "nobodies" in their chosen field, and sometimes are so emotionally blocked they may not even realize that they possess remarkable potential.

There are many psychological factors, both obvious and subtle, that compromise our ability to perform at our own top level. These factors include expectations of failure based on unrealistically high standards, fear of being watched or compared ("stage fright"), fear of others' resentments of our success, fear of injury, or memories of disappointments that make us shrink back from the crucial tests, among others. Few if any of us are free from such impediments. Meridian tapping can do a marvelous job in these areas. And when these mental/emotional impediments are cleared up — often quickly and simply — our natural talent can blossom to its fullest.

"Performance," we should remember, is not limited to something done on a sound stage or football field. The same rules that apply to athletes and actors apply to students, businesspeople, parents and community volunteers. We all have gifts we would like to maximize and skills that can be improved upon. Most of us also have performance barriers in some area or another that we'd like to be free from. For these we can now apply meridian tapping. The downside is practically nil, the upside is potentially huge.

Many of the issues related to performance are similar to those we discussed in the last chapter when we looked at fears. Often it is our fears and limiting self-talk that keep us "in the box" instead of "in the zone" and prevent us from excelling at our highest potential. We mentally set our performance "thermostat" at one fixed level and don't allow ourselves to expand beyond our "comfort zone". Gary waxes eloquent on this topic and has very kindly allowed me to reprint an article of his on this subject later in this chapter.

For the reasons just described, meridian tapping can be a brilliant addition to any skills training program. A wide range of professional athletes, musicians, coaches and everyday people have reported stunning breakthroughs in performance after only one or a few sessions of meridian tapping. These breakthroughs are happening in areas as diverse as:

- Public speaking
- Musical performance
- Sports
- Dance
- Academic skills
- Exam taking
- Sales
- Writer's block
- Business success

As with all uses of meridian tapping, the proof of the pudding is in the eating. *Your* eating in this case. Where would you like to optimize your performance and bring *your* highest natural talents to the foreground? The sky may be the limit here, as the following stories attest. Perhaps one of these real life accounts from Gary Craig's website will inspire you to create your own performance breakthrough in some brand new way.

"Magical Game" for Novice Bowler

To get things "rolling," here's a great meridian tapping story sent in by Arden Compton to Gary's site. It's told in Arden's own words *(with minor punctuation, wording and emphasis changes)*.

> Recently I took my family bowling. The bowling alley here in Brigham City was giving away a turkey to anyone who bowled 3 strikes in a row. So off we went to try our luck. Now, I am not a serious bowler; throughout my life, I have probably gone bowling about once a year... maybe less. I usually bowl somewhere between 100 and 120. If I get over 120, it is a good game for me, if I get into the 130s that's a *really* good game.

So, getting three strikes in a row wasn't likely — I might get two or three strikes in a game, but not in a row. In my first frame, I knocked over eight pins. Not bad. But I thought about how fun it would be to win a turkey and I decided to try some EFT. On my next turn, as I held the ball in my right hand, I tapped with my left hand on the face points and repeated in my mind, *"This fear of not making a strike."*

This time I bowled a spare, but got nine pins instead of eight. Each turn for the rest of the game, I went through the same tapping process. The next frame I bowled a strike! But on my two frames I bowled a spare — I needed three strikes in a row.

I was feeling pretty good about my game at this point; I was on track to an above-average score for me. Then the next frame I bowled a strike, and the following frame I bowled another strike! At this point I did a little tapping before my next turn — there was a little pressure because I was going for the turkey on this one. I tapped on *Fear of messing up the third strike… fear of not getting a strike.* I also tapped five seconds or so after I picked up my ball. And sure enough, I got a third strike!

I was so excited, I yelled loud enough for everyone in the bowling alley to hear me, "I won a turkey!" My wife and kids all gave me high fives. I ran over to the desk and had all the bowling alley employees give me a high five. There were some friends of mine several lanes down. I ran over to them and had them give me high fives. So, the next time I got the ball I tapped again, and I got another strike! Four in a row! And then I got another strike, and another one, and another one! Seven strikes in a row by the time the game ended. I bowled a 236, 100 points beyond what I thought would be a really good game.

> The statistical probability of me bowling seven strikes
> in a row has to be near zero. EFT really works! It calms
> us down, removes doubt and fear, which in turn allows
> us to perform at the level we are capable of. Try EFT
> for yourself and others — miracles can happen!

Note that Arden was already capable of bowling strikes, but not often or with great consistency. Tapping helped him gain the inner confidence to do this feat repeatedly, even under the exceptional pressure of the competition. This is the type of effect many athletes report with tapping.

College Scholarship Courtesy of Tapping

Marla Tabaka, an EFT practitioner, reports this story of a young athlete whose performance anxiety was holding him back. "Mark" was a football place-kicker with outstanding talent who had no problem nailing long field goals in practice and in games. But when it came to trying out for colleges, his performance shrunk to middling at best.

When Marla asked Mark to imagine himself kicking a football at an upcoming college camp he registered an anxiety intensity level of 9 on a scale of 0 to 10. He also exhibited a host of physical symptoms such as tingling in his legs, heaviness in his chest and redness in his ears.

What began to emerge, after some exploratory tapping work, was a fear Mark was carrying about being exposed to other players whose skills were as good as or better than his. Because of Mark's talent level, he had never encountered anyone with comparable skills to his on the local scene. As he imagined watching other players equal to or better than himself, he started questioning whether he deserved a scholarship and whether anyone would even notice him.

As Marla continued to work with Mark, using set-up phrases such as, "Even though I have more competition than I've ever bargained for…" and "This fear of the unexpected competition…," his anxiety began to *slowly* come down. That's when Mark began to uncover another hidden feeling — guilt at having been cocky in his junior year and not having practiced as hard as he should have. He felt a tremendous heaviness about this and believed he had let his team and his parents down.

Marla worked with him on clearing this. She used the image of a pile of "guilt bricks" pressing down on his chest. After several rounds of tapping away the bricks and forgiving himself for his 16-year-old immaturity, the redness in Mark's ears went away! He reported no more tingling in the legs and heaviness in the chest and said that his anxiety intensity had dropped to zero.

At the college camp, Mark tapped before taking the field, then performed beautifully. He was offered a scholarship to his second-choice college. He then vowed to try out for his number one college choice, which he had previously written off. His attitude had in fact changed on many levels. His meridian tapping sessions had seriously impacted Mark's life for the good.

Tapping and Public Speaking

Performance anxieties are not limited to athletes. One of the greatest fears reported by people of all ages, jobs, backgrounds and careers is speaking in public. Countless lives and careers are held in check due to reservations about talking in front of a group, *any* group, even speaking up at a business meeting with only a few people present. At the very least, many — perhaps *most* — of us would like to improve this skill. Here are a couple of quick examples of "instant" empowerment in this area through the use of tapping.

Nancy Rose Southern is a personal coach who sometimes officiates at weddings too since she is also an ordained minister. She reports a recent case of a bride whose anxiety about speaking in front of a crowd when she was to repeat her wedding vows was spoiling her anticipation of her special day. Nancy offered to do a tapping session with her and the groom before the wedding rehearsal. As the bride thought about saying her vows in front of 75-80 guests her anxiety level hit an 8-9 on a scale of 0 to 10. The groom's level was about a 3 or 4.

With a round of tapping, the groom easily came down to a 1, but the bride was a bit slower in responding. Nancy did several rounds of tapping with her, using slightly varied statements and approaches. During one of the rounds she reminded the bride that all the guests would be in attendance because they loved her.

The bride began silently crying. When Nancy asked her what the problem was, she said that thinking about all those guests coming to the wedding because they loved her felt so sweet it made her cry. Nancy offered to do more tapping, but the bride said "No, this feels like good crying."

Tapping, in the form of EFT, had worked to turn the situation around. During the actual wedding ceremony, both the bride and groom were relaxed and spoke their vows clearly and from their hearts. Nancy says that being able to offer EFT to couples to help them be more "present" for their weddings feels like a wonderful gift she can now offer as part of her officiating services.

A Second Public Speaking Story

Another impressive story about public speaking comes from Dawn Murray. She was running an EFT workshop and asked if anyone would like to work on their fear of public speaking. A teenaged girl named Melody — in the back row of course! — held up her hand in such a way as to block her face. When Dawn asked if she would come to the front of the room, she turned red and looked panicky, so Dawn did not push her.

Rather, Dawn did something interesting. She began tapping *her own* hand. She said, "Even though I am terrified to speak in front of people, I deeply and completely accept myself," and invited *everyone in the audience* to repeat the steps with her. They all tapped, as a group, on a few variations of this, ending with one round of the negative statement, "I am afraid to speak up in front of others in case I make a mistake and they laugh at me or ridicule me," followed by one round of the positive statement, "I comfortably and easily speak up for myself in a confident manner."

After this Dawn asked Melody how she felt.

Melody said she would need to have everyone in the room look at her to see if anything had changed. This statement alone was evidence of a remarkable change! Just minutes earlier she would have hidden her face or run out the door at such an idea.

Everyone turned to look at Melody and Dawn asked how she felt *now*. She said she would have to come to the front of the room to find out. She did so and Dawn asked her again how she felt. Melody replied that she'd have to *actually speak* to the audience to find out. When she did so she jokingly told the audience, "Go fly a kite!!" prompting a standing ovation from several of her friends in the audience.

Dawn explained to Melody that no one else had worked this magic *for* her. It was she, Melody, who had done the tapping and reclaimed her power. Melody really *got* it. She thanked Dawn and sat back down.

At the end of the evening Dawn asked if anyone would like to share their experience of that evening. Believe it or not it was Melody who first marched up to the front and spoke like a pro to the whole audience — she was calm, funny and open.

When Dawn followed up with her a few weeks later, she reported that she had confidently applied for a new job and was hired! Meridian tapping changes lives.

Tapping Helps Improve *Fishing*?!

"Try it on everything" is becoming the stock motto for using tapping. Here's an unusual example of what can happen when you heed that advice. It was reported to me by Hank Krol, a counselor at Stairways Behavioral Health, an outpatient mental health clinic in Erie, Pennsylvania.

"Claude" was a patient who sought help at the clinic following a prolonged hospitalization for major depression. When beginning to treat him, Hank wanted to demonstrate the efficacy of tapping right away so he had Claude tap for a shoulder and lower back pain. Claude experienced immediate relief and conceded that the tapping was effective.

When Claude returned a week later he asked Hank, quite out of the blue, if he thought tapping would "help me with my fishing."

Claude is semi-retired and one of his favorite pastimes is going down to the local creek where a number of experienced fishermen assemble daily. His girlfriend introduced him to fishing following his discharge from the hospital and he took to it, well, like a fish to water. Being somewhat of a perfectionist, he bought all the best equipment and carefully observed the other fishermen, making sure to use exactly the same bait they did, to fish in the same spots, and so forth. While he looked forward to his new hobby, it was also causing him substantial frustration.

The problem was, there were usually at least ten other fisherman lined up on the bank and, according to Claude, almost all of them would manage to catch large numbers of BIG steelhead trout each time they fished (Erie is the top city in the world for this variety of fish). Claude, on the other hand, would consistently leave at the end of the day with only a couple of small fish, if any, in his pail.

This was frustrating because to his knowledge he was doing nothing differently from the other fishermen, but rather following their procedures "to the letter." He recalls that he fished with minimal luck on at least fifteen to twenty occasions and did not experience a single successful day during that time.

Claude was persistent though. In fact, he was wearing his fishing boots at this session and preparing to return to the creek immediately after his appointment.

Hank responded to Claude's query about using meridian tapping for the problem by shrugging, "Let's try it." It is important to note that Hank did not have Claude address his poor fishing *results* as the problem when he was tapping — that is, he did not suggest tapping on, "Even though I'm a failure at fishing…" or similar statements. Instead he questioned Claude about his *emotional reactions* to the failure and asked Claude to tap only on his *feelings*.

Claude was able to identify three primary emotional reactions to this situation — "jealousy," "embarrassment," and a "lack of confidence" — emotions quite familiar to him in other situations as well. When he tapped on "embarrassment," his intensity was originally a "10" and after three rounds it had come down almost to 0. "Jealousy" was substantially reduced by the end of the session, and "lack of confidence" was similarly lessened. Claude was pleased with these results and marched out the door to test them at the creek.

When he returned for his next session he was incredulous.

He'd gone to the creek after his therapy session and found the other fishermen lined up, as usual, and pulling in fish after fish. Claude set up his fishing tackle and waited. But this time he didn't have to wait long. Within minutes he found himself, to his amazement, bringing in so many steelhead trout that he soon had caught more than he could possibly use — and they were big ones too!

This was the beginning of a new era. Claude systematically used tapping in the form of EFT each day before he fished, and each time that he tapped away his embarrassment and jealousy and lack of confidence he kept on having successes. A month or so later he reported that since beginning to use tapping he had experienced thirty to forty truly "good" fishing days, and only twelve days that were "not so good," a remarkable change from his earlier record. As of last report, his success at fishing continues, contributing greatly to his self-esteem.

Asked how he explains his extreme lack of success before he learned to tap, Claude says that he attributed it to "bad luck" and that he had been "unlucky" all of his life. But the fact that there was an immediate turnaround on the very day he commenced using tapping strongly suggests to him that "bad luck" really didn't have much to do with it. He says that when he taps on the three issues — embarrassment, jealousy, and lack of confidence — before he goes fishing (he does this religiously), he goes to the creek *expecting* to catch fish and that his lack of confidence is gone.

Now, under the guidance of Hank, Claude has begun using tapping for an even more basic issue — his lack of self esteem. He has noticed a marked improvement. Hank corroborates this, saying, "When [Claude] was in the hospital with severe depression his sense of self worth was a 0 on the 10-point scale. When he was discharged his sense of self worth rose to a 4... Now, after several months of treatment using meridian tapping with counseling for this problem, he rates his sense of self worth as 7... and, as a consequence, his depressive symptoms are now manageable for the first time."

Giving Claude a concrete place to start (i.e. his fishing) had helped him grow in ways that were now affecting every aspect of his life.

This is an intriguing story in many ways. Although we can speculate on many reasons for the positive outcome, actually none of us knows exactly how or why tapping worked to achieve its results from the standpoint of the *fish*. Is Claude now engaging in some new behavior when fishing that has turned the outcome around for him? If so, he is not aware of it. It is hard to imagine how confidence or lack thereof is conveyed to the fish. Many experienced fishermen, however, will tell you that confidence and expectation *do* make a huge difference in fishing. Why, we don't know.

One thing we are learning in this new era of energy science is that energies are not confined to the individual but can impact many other organisms and sometimes even inanimate objects (as in the incredible studies of the effects of thought on random number generators conducted by Robert Jahn, Dean of the School of Engineering at Princeton University). Reasoning from this perspective, one might wonder if Claude's relaxed and confident attitude about fishing is somehow being conveyed to the fish through means other than through the five senses. This would be similar in some ways to what happens during surrogate tapping (a process whereby we tap for someone else).

All of this is speculation, of course. I leave it to you to decipher The Mystery of Claude and the Steelhead Trout...

Using Tapping for Tone Deafness

At the beginning of the chapter, I stated that meridian tapping cannot give you skills you don't already possess. But we mustn't be too quick to decide that a talent is truly absent. Sometimes it's impossible to know what buried issues might be causing a person's natural abilities to be stifled. Here's a simple but fascinating example in which EFT was used to "produce" a talent that was well-hidden to all.

Arden Compton — our bowling friend — reports *(with minor punctuation, emphasis and wording changes):*

A few years ago my sister-in-law approached me and asked if I could help her 15-year-old son with his singing problem. He was tone-deaf. I frankly told her that I did not know because no one had ever come to me with that question before. I am always up for a challenge, though, so we decided to give it a try.

We started out by having her play a few notes on the piano and see if the boy could sing them. She hit middle C a few times but he was not able to get even close to hitting it. She tried a few other notes, but no matter what note she played, his voice was way off.

So, we started tapping for "this tone deaf problem." We tried reframing the problem a few different ways and then I muscle-tested him to see if there was an incident in his life that had initiated this problem. We determined that there was an event at age two where he was listening to his father sing, and he decided that for his father to love him, he needed to sing like his father. And his father was *not* singing well.

So, we tapped out for "this event" and "the belief that for father to love me I need to sing like father." Then we went back to the piano to see if there was any difference in his voice. Once again his mom hit middle C, but he was still off. She hit another note, and he didn't hit it, but his voice was moving around instead of just being way off. She hit a third note, and this time he started a little off, and then his voice slid to the right note. She hit a different note, and again his voice slid to the right note. It was a dramatic improvement.

A few days later he tried out for a play with a singing part in it, and he made it! I heard him sing a few months later at a family reunion. Someone had brought a karaoke setup, and people were taking turns singing along to different songs. When it came his turn I was stunned as I listened to him sing along with a very nice voice.

Here meridian tapping unearthed a hidden ability that had been entirely obscured as a result of Mark's previous history. He was now set free.

Tapping for Deep-Rooted Fears about Math

We can only speculate on how many ways tapping will eventually be used in education. I've had some excellent experiences using it this way myself, such as the time I used tapping to help my niece improve her driving skills, but I feel we've barely scratched the surface of its educational possibilities as yet.

Here is an encouraging story reported by a teacher by the name of Susitha.

> "16 year old 'Mara' (*name changed*) was an extremely hard worker in school but her performance in math was very poor. When I met [her], the thing that struck me was the sadness on her face. Mara told me she was good in all subjects except math. I asked her what her favorite subject was and she said 'chemistry.' I asked her about her feelings for math. She said her low marks make her sad and she 'knows' she will never be good at math."

Susitha and her student then did a few rounds of tapping for the sadness as Mara tried to recall an incident in the past when her feeling had been one of deep hurt regarding math. She suddenly remembered taking an important test years earlier in which she had scored 3 out of 10 correct answers and her former teacher had reprimanded her, proclaiming, "You will never be good at math!" Susitha, determined to help Mara undo the damage that had been done to her by the former one, had her tap to the following statements:

- "Even though the teacher said I will never be good at math, I choose to let that go. I choose to believe in myself and I completely forgive the teacher."
- "Even though I believed the teacher all these years I choose to believe in myself now. I forgive myself for believing the teacher and I love and accept myself.

- "Even though everyone was looking at me when the teacher said these words, I choose to let it go. I love and accept myself completely."

They then added some purely positive statements, such as, "I choose to like math now" and "I am good at math now." Susitha reminded her to tap on the positive statements every time she was working with math. Mara now reports that she "is making good progress and is finding math easy."

Gary Craig Looks at "The Comfort Zone"

Gary Craig, the founder of the EFT method or meridian tapping, was extensively and highly successfully engaged in athletics in his younger days. He has some intriguing and fruitful ideas about how we sometimes inadvertently hold ourselves back in our performance, whatever that may be, and how we can use tapping to stop doing that. Here, with Gary's permission, are excerpts from an article he wrote about this subject for his website (*edited slightly*):

> Using EFT for performance issues is one of my favorite topics. Not only is it highly effective but it is also fun and rewarding. Further, the results are often easy to recognize. While the principles in this article are applicable to ALL types of performance, I am going to emphasize mostly the sports area as a launching pad for these ideas.
>
> Over the years, I have played with and against hundreds of quality athletes and every one of them, regardless of how high they have risen in their sport, will tell you that they can "do better still." I've never seen an exception to that. Furthermore, they all agree that the main barrier to this better performance is due to the "mental part of the game." Their bodies are highly conditioned and their physical skills are second to none. Thus the difference between a superb day and a so-so one does not lie within their bodies. It resides

between their ears. This is fertile territory for a skilled EFT'er.

Experienced golfers, for example, know how to hit every shot perfectly. Their bodies have done it many times. They've hit perfect drives, perfect approach shots, perfect 15-foot putts… and so on (for an in-depth session on this see my work on golf with Clark on "The EFT Course" *DVDs* (see Resources Section). Despite this, golfers don't shoot perfect rounds and thus repeatedly fall below their optimum scores. They play a round of golf and hit a blend of both "perfect shots" and "not-so-perfect" shots and almost invariably end up scoring within their COMFORT ZONE.

The COMFORT ZONE is a critical concept within all performance pursuits. This is the mental place where an athlete subconsciously believes s/he "belongs." It is what keeps performance at its current level and, without properly addressing it, any improvements you develop for an athlete (or musician, or actor, etc.) are not likely to be lasting. Like a thermostat that keeps a room within a comfortable temperature range, our performance fluctuates within certain COMFORT ZONES. The COMFORT ZONE for golfers, for example, is reflected in their scores. Ask golfers what they shoot and they will answer with something like, "the mid 80s" or "the high 70s." This is their COMFORT ZONE. It is where they "belong" — even though they will tell you that they can do much better.

Interestingly, improving a specific part of a golfer's game (like putting) will not likely bring about an improved overall score. That's because other parts of the golfer's game will suffer in a manner that will allow the COMFORT ZONE (e.g. the mid-80s) to be maintained. Even if the golfer has a good day or a bad day and shoots out of their COMFORT ZONE, they will, on subsequent rounds, shoot once again where they "belong."

Let me give you a personal example. In high school I was a so-so basketball player. My only talent was my ability to jump like a kangaroo and gather rebounds. As a result I played center for our basketball team, a position normally given to the team's tallest player (someone 5 or 6 inches taller than me).

Upon getting a rebound I usually landed within five feet of the basket. Accordingly, you might think I was the team's leading scorer. After all, my shooting opportunities were from short range. But, alas, I only averaged two or three points per game because *I rarely took a shot.* Instead, I passed the ball out to one of the "shooters" on our team. If you think that is silly, you are right. Nonetheless, that's what I did... repeatedly.

Why? Because I had developed the self-talk in my head that rebounders are rebounders and that's it. Rebounders are not shooters. This is even more ridiculous when you consider the fact that I had the necessary hand-eye coordination to hit a speeding, curving baseball out of the park and had done so on many occasions. But somehow I had the belief that, because I was a rebounder, I was unable to put a ball into an oversized hoop from a mere five feet away.

Dumb.... really dumb.

But I can assure you that every performer, regardless of their caliber, carries around dozens of these dandy little dumbos and they aren't even aware they have them. Why? Because they have become routine beliefs AND no one has ever helped bring them to the surface so they can be EFT'd out of existence.

It would be nice if I could give you a nice clean list of all of these specific impediments to performance, together with a neat and precise recipe for handling each of them. But, alas, a list of these endless comedies would stretch from here to the middle of the Cosmos. However, with a little creativity and detective work you can soon uncover these hidden thieves.

Here are some guidelines...

1. Often there is a disguised "penalty" for performing to one's maximum. Perhaps one thinks that outperforming one's father/mother/brother/sister will result in a loss of their love. Or maybe they think that if they achieve that new level, they will be expected to maintain it (which they erroneously think will require too much effort). There are many potential penalties. Dig for them. You will often uncover treasure chests filled with ripe issues that need resolution.

2. Sometimes there is a limiting emotional response to a competitor or to a certain auditorium, academic subject, golf course, etc. I recall many times when a certain pitcher... or golf hole... or football stadium was "bigger than me." There was something about the circumstances that "had my number." The resulting self doubts, of course, affected my play.

3. Many performers focus on what they do well and let slide other aspects of their performance that "aren't as important." However, mastering those other "little things" adds measurably to the overall performance.

Quality detective work will almost always find the *specific events* in the past that are showing up as limits in performance and, once found, EFT is highly likely to collapse them. The result, of course, is a new level of Emotional Freedom that manifests as better scores, better grades, better acting, better writing... and happier people.

Well said, Gary. Thanks for letting me include this article.

In the next chapter we'll take a look at how tapping can help with one of the most stubborn issues of our times: weight loss.

Tapping "Choices" to Enhance Performance

Even though I'm worried about this upcoming event *(this new challenge, how I'll do, etc.)*...

...I choose to be calm and confident.

...I choose to remember how well I did when I *(insert here any situation where you performed any task whatsoever successfully and felt good about it).*

...I choose to feel like *(insert here the name of your hero or heroine, or the star you would like to be like)* as I play the game *("give the speech", etc.)*

At our clinic we are presently using meridian tapping to help patients overcome negative emotions that undermine health, and to eliminate many forms of pain... We also use it to reduce food cravings that can sabotage healthy eating programs, and to implement positive life goals to support optimal health and well being... Tapping is now a major component of our treatment program.*

Dr. Joseph Mercola
Director, Optimal Wellness Center
Founder/Host, www.mercola.com

Tapping belongs to everyone who uses it, in that sense it is "universal".

*Quote by Dr. Joseph Mercola, one of the experts in the movie, *The Tapping Solution*.

Chapter 12

Try Tapping to Improve Weight Loss

One of the most frustrating challenges of modern life seems to be losing weight and keeping it off. A multi-billion-dollar industry has sprung up around exploiting this problem. Many of us have purchased hundreds, even thousands of dollars' worth of diet books, diet equipment, diet workshops or diet club memberships and most of it is gathering dust.

Every year some new diet sweeps the world, claiming to be the real thing. It tells us that it will succeed where others have failed. Some of them even work. For a while. Six months or a year later, though, the bathroom scale is tipping into the red zone again.

What is the problem here?

Actually, the biggest reason diets don't work is that they focus on food and food is *not* the issue. That's right. *Food is not the issue.* The real cause of our weight epidemic stems from that mysterious impulse that makes us get off the couch, forty-five minutes after a satisfying meal, and head for the fridge to have a look around. Until we solve the problem at *that* level, we're never going to get very far with diets. The root cause of overeating is not the food, it's the emotions underlying our compulsion to eat.

This is where tapping comes in. It is giving thousands of people a new and effective tool to free them from the underlying causes of overeating, often for the first time in their lives.

You've probably heard the term "emotional overeating" and have a sense of what it means. Clearly, when a person is tearing into his third bag of potato chips, something more than *survival* needs is at work. The problem is that, up until now, there hasn't been a quick, powerful and inexpensive way to address the emotional aspect of eating. Tapping fills that void.

Before we look at some specific emotions that contribute to overeating, let's take a very general look at where the problem arises from. (This is described in greater detail in the E-book, *The Key to Successful Weight Loss*, written by Dr. Carol Look, Dr. Sandra Radomski and myself and included as part of the meridian tapping computer program of the same name.)

Overeating, it seems, may very well stem from the fact that life is changing faster than biophysical evolution can keep up! You see, just a very, very short time ago — from an evolutionary standpoint — our species did not have such modern conveniences as supermarkets, freezers, salaries and checking accounts. So anytime the food supply ran low, our survival was under threat. Literally. Lack of food triggered an immediate signal to our bodies that we were in danger. Release the adrenalin! Save yourself!

Correspondingly, the feeling of a full stomach was a signal of biological comfort and safety — a bodily message that no matter what happens in the near future, I know I can survive. So I can relax for a while.

Unfortunately, our instincts haven't had a chance to catch up with the reality of modern life, where we no longer have to hunt or gather or fight off wild scavengers. We still equate a feeling of being full with a sense of, "I'm safe!"

What happens is that this feeling of "safety" we get from food is applied to a host of "threatening" emotions that have nothing to do with our physical survival. Eating makes us feel good and makes bad emotions go away. One theory about why carbohydrates, in particular, feel so comforting (as in "comfort foods") is that the rapid rise in blood sugar they give us translates to a physical feeling that we have been miraculously "saved" from starvation. We're out of danger.

This physical feeling of being saved is a balm we apply whenever *any* "dangerous" feeling — anger, anxiety, loneliness, shame, deprivation — threatens to take us over. And here's the interesting twist. If we grab for a comforting food *fast* enough, we can often avoid consciously feeling that unpleasant emotion in the first place.

Food can act so efficiently to mask an unwelcome feeling that we may not even recognize the connection between the feeling and our desire for the food. And that's why the emotional aspect of overeating often remains unrecognized by us. In a sense, we're solving the problem before it occurs. So we don't witness it. And the price we're paying is that we're eating ourselves to death.

Researchers estimate that 95 percent of diets fail because most diet and exercise programs do not address the root problem — emotional overeating.

Now at last, however, there is a simple and universally available tool we can use to address the troubling emotions themselves. Meridian tapping allows us to do what diets can't do — tackle the root of the issue.

The fact is that emotions can't harm us, we just think they can. When we learn to be at peace with whatever emotions come up, rather than "running" from them as if they were threats, we can accept them and move through them quickly. We no longer have to anesthetize or protect ourselves against them. Tapping helps us get to this point.

Anger as a Trigger for Overeating

Anger is an emotion that often triggers a compulsive need to eat, especially if we feel we *can't* or *shouldn't* express that anger for one reason or another. Why does eating help with anger? Well, one very basic reason is that the act of *biting* itself is a very primitive way of channeling rage. On an animal level we literally want to bite the enemy. Instead we sink our teeth into a tough bagel or a fistful of crunchy cheese curls! The acting of biting combined with the calming biochemical effect of the food disperses the angry impulse. Tension resolved. At least for the moment.

Another reason we apply food to anger is that being angry may feel dangerous to us. We may be afraid of what will happen if we express this (perfectly natural) emotion so we opt for the "safety" of food to ward off the feeling of danger that anger causes.

There are many reasons why anger can trigger emotional overeating. The good news is that we don't need to spend years in therapy to root these reasons out (although therapy can often help). We can simply apply tapping and resolve the problem in a much more immediate way.

Here's a story by my colleague and good friend Carol Look (*edited here*) about how she used meridian tapping to successfully treat an "angry overeater" who had multiple issues.

> "Ann" was referred to me for weight loss by her back pain doctor who had recently heard of meridian tapping. The doctor felt the excess weight was a contributing factor for her overall pain and general health condition.
>
> Ann said she was overweight most of her life, and sometimes used food to "stick it to" her mother. She used food when she was irritated by her mother and to show that she was "in charge." She understood how this backfired, however, but was unable to stop using food in this way when feeling angry or resentful. "I eat to squash the turmoil" is how she put it.
>
> Chronically angry at her mother, Ann felt as if she were the adult in the relationship. Essentially she was hungry for basic love and acceptance from her mother and never felt heard or understood.

These feelings had been carried over into her marriage as well. Sensing the anger that was driving much of Ann's overeating, Carol had her tap for several different issues with set-up phrases such as:

- For her mother issues − "Even though my mother doesn't even like me, I completely like and accept myself." "Even though my mother doesn't think I'm good enough, I choose to believe I'm lovable and good enough."

- For her health issues — "Even though I'm angry that no one knows what I've been through, I accept and love myself." "Even though I feel enraged by my pain, I deeply and completely accept myself."
- For her marriage issues — "Even though I feel angry when he doesn't listen to me, I choose to listen to myself." "Even though I feel terribly frustrated because I'm starving for love and affection, I want to feel comforted anyway." "Even though I feel rejected and it feels painful, I deeply and completely accept myself."

Ann continued to tap between sessions with Carol and soon began reporting remarkable transformations. According to Carol:

> She isn't bothered by her mother anymore and feels more at peace with what she didn't experience emotionally as a child. "Food isn't as central in my life anymore… I eat moderately and am more conscious of when I'm full and what I need. I enjoy not cramming food down my throat anymore." She still eats her favorite foods but has a new awareness about what her body needs. "I no longer have to eat to fill the starvation I feel."
>
> Ann used to binge on cookies and sweets in the afternoon. Now she takes that time to be by herself, read, think about her feelings, and tap. She acknowledges that neither her mother nor her husband have changed in any way, however, she feels confident she can identify and process all of her feelings in relationship to both of them. Her pain is much better, and she continues to seek professional medical help for long-term ailments.
>
> Ann has lost 25 pounds and feels confident that she will make it through the holidays with ease.

Anxiety and Food

Anyone who has ever experienced anxiety knows how uncomfortable and distressing it can feel. Anxiety hurts. It might best be defined as a state of extreme unease brought on by the *anticipation* of some future circumstance, real or imagined. One could almost call anxiety "fear of the future."

Anxiety triggers many of the same bodily reactions as a "real" threat to our safety does, even though no physical threat is present. We human beings tend to get anxious about a host of things that do not directly threaten our safety — taking an exam, attending an important meeting, speaking in public, having a confrontation with a boss or loved one... The causes are innumerable. The symptoms can include dry mouth, sweaty palms, increased heartbeat, shakiness in the body and pressure in the chest.

Anxiety generally arises out of situations where we feel that we *lack control* of the outcome. It is easy to see, then, why we often seek to remedy the situation through food. Food and drink give us an immediate way to *regain* control, at least on a superficial level. We eat the chocolate bar or the doughnut and we instantly create that sense of physical safety and comfort I described above.

But, of course, we're not really addressing the root of the anxiety, so it never gets resolved. It's like taking painkillers for a repeating toothache, rather than going to the dentist.

Tapping lets us intercede with the root cause by altering the energy patterns that are directly producing the feelings of fear. When we change the fear or nervousness itself, we no longer have to lunge for the Oreo cookies.

Here's a real-life example of tapping being used for anxiety (*edited slightly*), taken from our E-book, *The Key to Successful Weight Loss*.

> Doug's job included weekly public speaking in front of his whole department and boss. As he would approach the podium, he would sweat more than usual, feel a strange out-of-body sensation and experience light-headedness. While he always managed to get through

these speeches, he was sure everyone noticed how anxious he was. He often feared he would be fired because of this.

After Doug got through these ordeals, he had a ritual — he indulged in binge eating. Although he could still hide some of the extra pounds, he knew that eating enough food for three adult males was not normal. The problem was, Doug ate so fast and in such a trance state, he barely knew what was happening.

Using tapping, Doug set to work first to deal with his anxiety about the speeches. After just a couple of sessions of tapping on this, he was able to approach the podium with excitement, rather than anxiety.* He then tapped some more on this issue and found that he was learning how to lower his voice and slow down his words. When he did this he found himself having a more realistic and positive perception of the job he performed when he was talking.

At first, he still had the habit of overeating in solitude after one of these events. He then used tapping for this habit, and was able to relax and enjoy himself after his speeches and treat himself to a normal meal instead.

He soon noticed other times he ate more food than necessary. Working consistently with the EFT form of meridian tapping, he was eventually able to calm the inner turmoil that was affecting his confidence level, and then was able to shed the extra pounds quite easily. More importantly, he felt proud instead of ashamed of his behavior when speaking in public.

---

* It's interesting to note that many of the feelings and symptoms we attribute to anxiety are the same as those we attribute to excitement. Often it is only the interpretation of the event — positive vs. negative — that causes us to categorize the feelings as good or bad.

Eating Shame Away

Shame is another negative emotion that we often try to tamp down with food. Shame is a dreadful feeling. When we feel ashamed, we want to disappear into the woodwork or hide under the furniture. We feel we aren't good enough to share the public oxygen supply and don't deserve people's time or positive attention. Food provides us with the comfort we feel unable to glean from others or provide for ourselves.

But it is far more productive to *change* the shame than to gloss it over with a "food fix."

Shame is not a helpful emotion if we want to move our lives in any kind of positive direction, such as losing weight. Being able to accept ourselves as we are, even with our overweight bodies and bad eating habits, is an important first step toward successful weight loss.

Tapping is very useful in this regard. As you learn to be kind to yourself, to accept yourself and forgive yourself for whatever past "crimes" you feel you have committed, you will find yourself much more willing and able to let go of comfort foods. You simply won't need to tranquilize yourself anymore! And then you can begin eating the way you consciously choose.

Tapping helps you build a more positive, loving and accepting attitude about yourself. And these changes can start to be felt almost immediately once you find the tapping words and set-up phrases that work for you.

Here's a One-Minute Wonder reported by Kathleen Sales on Gary Craig's web site (*edited slightly*). It deals with a memory of shame that was getting in the way of weight loss.

> My client wanted to not only lose weight but also to find a way to maintain that weight loss. She had tried every program under the sun and had been successful at losing weight, but always seemed to gain it back and then some.
>
> I explained to her that we could definitely work on the issue of weight and maintenance but that we would also need to focus on emotional issues affecting her life since typically the issue of excess weight is not about

the food at all. She agreed to the commitment and we were on our way.

I asked the typical questions about weight: How long have you had a weight problem? When did you first recognize that you had a weight problem? Do others in your family struggle with weight?

All of a sudden, her face began to tense up as she spoke of her Godmother who had basically tortured her as a young girl. Every weekend her family would make a trip to visit their Godparents and whenever no one was watching her Godmother would say to her, "God, you're fat!" Keep in mind, this was a girl about 6 or 7. This went on until the age of 9 or 10.

These words echoing in her head brought great sadness and anger to the surface so this is where we began. I asked her what her intensity rating was regarding this issue and she said "Ohhhh, it's a 10 definitely!" I had her close her eyes and repeat after me:

- "Even though I hear these cruel words *God, you're fat...* I deeply and completely love and accept myself."
- "Even though Claire's (*not her real name*) cruel words echo loudly *God, you're fat...* I deeply and completely accept myself and my body."
- "Even though I hear Claire's hurtful, mean and cruel words *God, you're fat...* I completely love and accept myself anyway."

We then tapped on the following,

- God, you're fat!
- Those hateful cruel words *God, you're fat.*
- Claire's voice echoing *God, you're fat.*
- Those cruel, cruel words echoing inside of me *God, you're fat.*

After some more tapping that involved the Nine Gamut spot — part of the EFT and TFT "long version" — and then doing some more clearing rounds, Kathleen reports:

> I asked her to remain with her eyes closed and go inside to see what was there. She felt a sense of calm. Her face had definitely lightened up and showed the results of the tapping. I then asked her to repeat the words "God, you're fat!" to see if anything came up. She did and smiled. "They're just words, they have no effect on me whatsoever. Claire is gone!"

> At our next session I asked her to again repeat the words, "God, you're fat!" and absolutely nothing occurred. Just a smile and a shake of the head. During the course of our work together, we found another person that needed to be "let go of" and when that surfaced my client said, "Oh goody, are we going to be able to make him disappear just like we did Claire?" We did and it was another incredible result of EFT.

Other Reasons for Emotional Overeating

Reasons for emotional overeating could fill a book of their own. Other common negative emotions we often try to nullify through food include:

- Sadness
- Loneliness
- Depression
- Boredom
- Guilt
- Frustration
- Discouragement

Tapping can be used to address all of these. The important thing is to pay attention to when and under what circumstances you overeat so that you can begin to identify which emotions are coming into play. Then come up with the appropriate phrases to use in your tapping sessions.

Some other common reasons for overeating include:

- **Rebelliousness** — Many of us tire of trying to "be good" all the time and play our life roles so perfectly. One common way to regain a feeling of freedom and independence is to overeat wildly. Tapping, however, can help us find authentic emotional freedom without physically harming ourselves in the process.

- **"I deserve a treat today!"** — Sometimes we work so hard and stretch ourselves so thin, we just want to be rewarded. Though overeating can seem like a reward, tapping can help us establish ways to genuinely reward ourselves — ways that are healthy, satisfying and life-enhancing, such as yoga, dancing, nature walks, or playing an instrument for fun. The possibilities are endless!

- **Family Eating Patterns** — Our early family patterns of eating affect us in ways of which we are often unaware. Perhaps your parents, for example, fought at the dinner table so you learned to wolf your food down so as to quickly make your getaway. Or maybe you were given food every time you were sad. These habits tend to carry into adulthood. Tapping can help us in our conscious effort to develop new and healthily adaptive habits.

- **Fear of the Consequences of Weight Loss** — Yes, there can be "scary" consequences for losing weight. If you slim down you might suddenly attract romantic attention you're not prepared for. Or maybe you'll make a sibling or friend jealous. These considerations often keep the overeating machine going. Once you identify a fear such as these, you can target it with tapping.

- **Social Overeating** — Some of us manage the munching just fine when we're alone, but whenever we're with other people — or certain other people — the brakes are off. Insecurities, social discomfort, anxieties over the role we are expected to play — all of these factors can prompt us to reach for the chemical comfort of food. Tapping wonderfully addresses social anxieties and can solve the problem of social overeating at its roots.

- **Overeating "Triggers"** — Certain situations, places or times of day can trigger compulsive eating — sitting in front of the television, visiting parents, going on vacation, etc. Once you become consciously aware of your habitual triggers, you can use tapping to neutralize them.

Some User Feedback on Tapping for Weight Loss

The incredible thing about using tapping for weight loss is that it really works. For many, many people. That means we no longer have to struggle though endless cycles of dieting and regaining weight and all of the self-recrimination that comes along with it. In fact, I envision the day, not far into the future, when no one will dream of tackling a weight loss program without leveraging the strengths of Energy Psychology, particularly meridian tapping. Here are a few comments about this I've collected on my web site.

> My husband and I both had a longstanding sugar addiction. Because we'd heard that meridian tapping can be used to reduce addictive cravings, we decided to try EFT for this, although we doubted it would do much good. So we tapped daily for a short while for "these sugar cravings." The results were so marvelous we could scarcely believe it! I lost 15 pounds after that without really consciously changing anything. I simply wasn't at the mercy of my craving anymore. We both still eat sugar, but WE decide when we really want it and how much we really need, we don't feel we HAVE to have it... If I could, I would recommend EFT to everyone I see. — **Karen Fitch, Stay at Home Mom**

> At our clinic we are presently using meridian tapping to help patients overcome negative emotions that undermine health, and to eliminate many forms of

pain... We also use it to reduce food cravings that can sabotage healthy eating programs, and to implement positive life goals to support optimal health and well being... Tapping is now a major component of our treatment program. **– Dr. Joseph Mercola, Director, Optimal Wellness Center, Chicago, Illinois**

I was addicted to carbs and have been on a diet most of my life. Never in my wildest dreams did I think tapping would work for me. To my amazement it almost immediately helped me feel in control of myself... I lost my cravings. I lost the extra pounds and kept them off... most importantly, I didn't feel deprived... **– Kathy Hornbach , Full-time Mom**

Shortly after I started using meridian tapping an incredible thing happened. I'm 50 pounds overweight and I've tried for years to lose some of that weight with no success at all. Well, after about a week of using [EFT] and only intensively for 2 to 3 days of that week, I had lost 5 pounds! I had done nothing at all differently and was on no diet. Since then I've been running around the countryside like a maniac and haven't put back any of that loss. I think tapping is an amazing tool!" **– Therese Bower, Massage Therapist**

If you have tried to lose weight by dieting and have been unsuccessful, or have repeatedly put the pounds back on, I can't encourage you strongly enough to give meridian tapping a try. If you feel you need professional help with your weight loss program, call a meridian tapping practitioner in your area (see Finding a Practitioner Section in back of book). Often only one or a few short sessions are all that is needed to start you down the path to real and lasting success. Failure at weight loss need no longer be a standard expectation.

Tapping "Choices" for Weight Loss

Even though I crave this food...

> ...I choose to pass it up for now.

> ...I choose to remember my commitment to myself.

> ...I choose to find other ways to handle my anxiety *(anger, distress etc.)*.

> ...I choose to keep my goal weight constantly in mind.

> ...I choose to be a good friend to myself.

When there's pain in the body, that's a signal something is not in harmony with the laws of the universe...*

Bob Proctor
Success Mentor
Featured in "The Secret"

Tapping restores harmony and balance to our energy systems — an indirect attack on all pain.

*Quote from Bob Proctor in the movie, *The Tapping Solution.*

Chapter 13

Try Tapping for Physical Conditions and Pain

The widespread use of meridian tapping for dealing with pain that is now being reported might be expected when we consider that the most prevalent use of acupuncture in Western countries is for pain control (anesthesia). As a direct heir to acupuncture, tapping uses many of the same principles as acupuncture. It's not surprising, then, that tapping can also be extremely effective for pain relief.

According to acupuncture theory, physical trauma can cause a major disruption in the body's bio-energy system. Fortunately, tapping can "reroute" and calm down that energy disruption easily, often dramatically lessening pain or eliminating it entirely. The results of using tapping for pain are often described as "amazing," "unbelievable," "astonishing." Sometimes the pain is gone so suddenly, the sufferer forgets all about it or attributes the relief to another cause.

A remarkable side benefit of its powerful pain reducing properties is tapping's apparent healing effects on the source of the pain — the underlying condition. There is much clinical evidence to show that if a person uses meridian tapping daily as a self-treatment for the pain or injury, *actual healing* of the underlying condition often occurs. We see the same happen with acupuncture. One acupuncture treatment may not do the trick, but a *series* of treatments can sometimes make a dramatic difference in the underlying condition.

One reason tapping may be so effective with pain and physical conditions may be due to the fact that for many, even most, medical conditions, there is an underlying emotional condition which is presently unresolved. It is a well-established medical fact that every emotion we have triggers a dizzying array of chemicals in the body. Joyous emotions produce healing chemicals while negative emotions dump disease-causing chemicals into our systems.

It is not a great stretch, therefore, to see that a persistent negative emotional state can generate persistent illness and pain.

Currently, drugs are our pain treatment of choice in the West.

"Drugs," however, as Gary Craig points out, "tend to temporarily help the chemical causes of pain but they have limited ability to reduce any long term underlying emotional causes. Tapping, on the other hand, collapses these emotional causes and that is why long term pain relief is often achieved."

It is an undeniable fact that many serious illnesses have responded to meridian tapping. One explanation of this is that a *combination* of the intrinsic healing properties of meridian-based treatment *and* the fact that tapping handles the emotional factors that can underlie an illness, results in the highly beneficial effects we see when tapping is applied to pain.

Meridian tapping has been reported to bring relief for such a wide array of physical problems and their resulting pain that it is impossible to mention them all here. A very partial list includes:

- Toothache
- Back pain and injury
- Burns
- Insect stings
- Ligament injuries
- Muscle cramps
- Injuries due to accident
- Arthritis
- Spinal misalignment
- Urinary problems
- Infections
- Sore throat

- Carpal Tunnel Syndrome
- Frozen shoulder
- And many others.

The list goes on and on. While we must caution that tapping should not be used in place of medical treatment for serious conditions, it is now clear that it can be an extraordinary adjunct to traditional Western treatments. For minor conditions, conditions resistant to treatment, and/or persistent pain stemming from previously treated conditions, tapping alone can, and often does, bring spectacular results.

The following stories will give you just a small taste of the benefits currently being reported by applying tapping to physical conditions and pain.

How I Saved "Tech Support" from a Toothache

What is one of the most common types of pain almost all of us experience at some point in our lives? Toothaches! A toothache can quickly ratchet up to a 10 on the pain scale. And when it does, it can eclipse all other thoughts. You might assume that pain this acute and extreme would not respond to a technique as "soft" as meridian tapping. However, toothache relief, is one of the most frequent benefits reported from the use of tapping. Here's an experience I myself had recently.

My computer had had a meltdown (again!) and was pretty nearly nonfunctional. After much time waiting on hold I had finally reached a friendly and knowledgeable tech support person. No sooner had I experienced the relief of finding someone who seemed to know how to fix my problem than he interrupted our session by announcing, "I'm sorry, but I'm not sure I can continue with this. I have such a bad pain in my wisdom tooth, I think I may have to quit for the day."

Before he could get off the phone, I quickly informed him that I am a specialist in stress management and asked him if he would be willing to try a simple tapping technique based on acupuncture that is often very effective for tooth pain. "I'd try *anything*!" was his answer.

I then instructed him where to tap and had him repeat the phrase, "Even though I have this severe pain, I choose to have my jaw and teeth feel normal and comfortable." The Choices Method, which I was employing here, seemed the ideal approach to use with a stranger whom I'd just met on the phone because sometimes the self-acceptance statements in the traditional form of EFT can throw off skeptics and newcomers.

I then led him through one entire tapping sequence. After a complete round, when I asked him to check his wisdom tooth pain, he said with a note of surprise in his voice, "Well — actually it's better."

I then led him through another round of tapping at the end of which I again inquired about the pain intensity. There was a several-second silence at the other end of the phone. Then I heard him say, in an incredulous tone, "This is awesome! It's *much* better." His pain was now about a 3 on the 0 to 10 point scale of intensity.

We did one more round of tapping, which I explained to him was so that we could be sure his pain relief had a good chance of lasting. He tapped a round once more at my request and at the end of it he said about the pain, "I can hardly notice it now" and exclaimed once more, "This is awesome!"

He felt he didn't need any more tapping and cheerfully resumed his tech support session with me (to my relief!). A half hour later, when he had completely resolved my computer problem — he was an excellent technician — he was preparing to wind up the call and I said, "Just to check on where you're at, how does your wisdom tooth feel now?"

"To tell you the truth," he answered rather apologetically, "I'd forgotten about it." This is a familiar response of someone who has been doing meridian tapping. I instructed him how to tap at home if he needed it again, and that ended the incident. He simply muttered, "Awesome..." again, as he put down the phone.

Tapping Eliminates a Serious Sore Throat

You may have experimented with certain "New Age" healing or self-improvement techniques. Typically, when they work, the technique is given the credit, but when they fail, YOU are given the blame. "You didn't believe enough." "You had a negative attitude." "You sabotaged the treatment." etc.

An outstanding thing about tapping, as I've said in this book, is that it works regardless of your views toward it. All that is really required is that you be open enough to try it. Skeptics are not "punished" for their non-belief. They too get results!

Of course, the more you tap and experience its benefits, the more "sold" you become on the method. You can now trust it. But you are not required to believe in it — why would you be? — your first time out of the starting gate. Or *ever* for that matter. That's why we confidently offer the invitation, "*Try* it on everything." You can view it simply as an experiment and just see what happens!

Here's a story *(edited slightly)* that illustrates this point. It was sent in to Gary's site from an Australian skeptic-turned-"convert" named Jann Barry:

> Three years back I had a visit from a friend. Just as she was leaving she reached into the car, handed me a small book, and said, "Oh here, I forgot to give you this. I'm sure you'll find it interesting as you're into all this weird stuff." Don't you just LOVE your friends?

> The book was *Pocket Guide to Emotional Freedom* by Steve Wells and David Lake.

> Later that day I was driving a cold-infected friend to town when she was overcome with a coughing, sneezing fit. All I could think was that the interior of the car was now wall to wall microbes and that no matter how many positive affirmations I fed my immune system it was a "done deal" that I would get her cold.

> That night I took the book to bed with me. I can't remember how far in I got but when it started talking about tapping on bits of the body and repeating statements I put the book down in disgust! "I don't

think so!" I said in disbelief and snapped off the light. The concept was too weird — even for me!

Around 4 a.m. I was awoken with THE mother of all sore throats. On a scale of 0-10, I was a 25 heading for 100. I put on the light and just sat there thinking, "bloody hell (we Australians tend to say this a lot)."

Just then my eyes rested on the book. Well, I thought, what have I got to lose? So, picking it up, I followed the bouncing ball so to speak.

First focus on the problem — well THAT was easy. Next, rate the problem on a scale of 1-10. Yep, a good 100. Now tap here 3 times whilst stating the problem. O.K. "Even though I have this bloody sore throat that feels like I swallowed a bunch of razorblades..." Now tap here and here and here, etc.

What now? Rate the problem again! Dear God, this meant I had to swallow. I sat there gathering my courage and then, very tentatively, I swallowed. Then I swallowed again and NOTHING! It was completely gone. Not just a *bit* better, not just moved to the other side of the throat but totally gone.

I did what any Newbie would do. I said to myself that I actually didn't have a sore throat, that I must have dreamt it. Well, the reality was I *knew* I'd had it. I thought, "Well I'll sit here for 5-10 minutes and it'll be back." Fifteen minutes later, no sore throat so I turned off the light and went to sleep.

Next morning as my eyes flicked open my first thought was, "Bet it's back now." But it wasn't and neither did I get the cold! So there I was, this Grade A Skeptic, following a technique I absolutely didn't believe in, who had become in that one moment totally and absolutely hooked.

Thumb Pain Arrested

Just as you are not required to have faith in tapping in order for it to lessen your pain, you are not required to assume any particular attitude while tapping either. For example, you don't even need to be unnecessarily serious. Here's a story *(edited slightly)* by John Fletcher, who successfully taught meridian tapping to an injured workman in his home, even though both of them approached the whole thing rather loosely and irreverently.

John and his wife had recently been introduced to EFT and had used it to clear up a headache of hers. John tells this story:

> A couple of days later we had workmen redoing our bathroom. One was removing pipes with a reticular saw when he dropped the saw and held his hand up to his face, yelling out in pain. I thought he had seriously cut his hand. When I asked what happened, he said he had injured his thumb the day before when he got hit with a horseshoe. He said he didn't think it was broken but it was bruised and swollen. He said he wasn't sure if he was going to be able to work today because it hurt so badly.
>
> I asked him if wanted me to take him to the hospital. He said, "No, it will be okay," but it was obvious he was in pain. So I just blurted out, "Billy, would you be interested in trying this amazing thing called tapping?" I explained what I understood about moving energy around and accepting yourself. I laughed, saying it didn't make a whole lot of sense to me but that it worked with my wife and others I saw on these DVDs.
>
> My explanation took less than 30 seconds and he said, "Yeah, I'll try it, it can't hurt." I asked him the pain level on a 0 to 10 scale. He said it was about an 8 or 9. I had him tap and say out loud that even though he had this real sore thumb he totally accepted himself.

We both laughed out loud at how ridiculous this was. But I continued on in a very lighthearted way and told him to say "sore thumb" as he tapped on all the points I saw on the DVD. He smiled with a look that said, "I can't believe I'm doing this," but announced in disbelief that the pain was a lot less. Still half-laughing, I asked, "How much less on the scale?"

"About a 3," he said.

I was getting excited. We tapped some more on the "remaining pain." We both were still next to laughter. I asked him how it was now. "A zero," he yelled. Neither of us could believe what had happened. I followed him downstairs and listened in amazement when he told his work partner that his thumb didn't hurt any more. We looked at each other and laughed again.

Well... I guess EFT *is* pretty funny, especially when you're used to long healing periods and high medical bills!

Tapping Clears Longstanding Back Pain and Restores Quality of Life

Sometimes we forget how pain robs our lives of quality and freedom. We become used to living with it and making the reduced choices that the pain dictates. Often there are underlying emotional issues that never get addressed because our focus is always on the pain itself. Here is a story of a man who recovered from debilitating back pain by using meridian tapping and also recovered his *life* in the process.

Graham Batchelor runs a sports injury clinic. One day he was visited by a 45-year-old man who had suffered a major injury to his lower back. After spending six months in the hospital and another two years in a wheelchair, the man had begun walking with two crutches but could only cover about 100 feet before becoming exhausted. He was on powerful painkillers and moved with a very lopsided posture. Just the effort to get to the appointment had completely worn him out. He could barely climb onto the treatment couch.

Graham had only just begun to learn tapping in the form of EFT, but he had the sense that this patient might be able to benefit. Upon talking to the man, it became evident that he was suffering a great deal of guilt over his inability to help his wife when she'd recently undergone major surgery. He was also suffering a lot of self-recrimination due to the fact that he had lost his earning power. When Graham asked him to rate his quality of life on a scale of 1 to 10, he gave it a 2. But he did agree to try tapping. Graham took him through a standard set-up procedure, using phrases such as:

"Even though I have this serious injury…"

"Even though I could not help my wife in her time of urgent need…"

"Even though I can no longer support my family…"

By the time they reached the collarbone point, Graham says:

…he began sobbing, his breathing became labored and his lower body began twitching. We stopped and I explained that I thought he was going through a very strong emotional release. He gradually regained composure and we carried on.

At the end of the second round he requested that we continue, indicating he felt much better emotionally and his pain was reducing. After the third round I prepared to help him off the couch. Amazingly, he stood up by himself and, using only one stick, began walking around the treatment room.

I advised him not to be too adventurous and just take things a little easy. With tears of happiness in his eyes he said he could not thank me enough. I explained that tapping and himself were the healers and I was only a channel.

Before leaving the office, the patient told Graham that his quality of life had already shot up to 9 out of 10 and that he could not wait to get home. Three days after the treatment, both he and wife incredulously reported that they could not believe his recovery.

Amputation Averted Through Tapping

As I pointed out at the beginning of the chapter, one of the most exciting developments using meridian tapping on the medical front is that it is not just relieving pain, but is often clearing up actual medical conditions at the same time. Patients are *getting* better, not just *feeling* better. Here is a dramatic case of a man who avoided life-altering surgery through the use of meridian tapping.

Jan Scholtes works in the Physiotherapy Department of a hospital in Holland where "Hans" (not his real name) was an outpatient who had long been suffering from severely impaired circulation in his legs. He had already undergone five ineffective bypass operations and was experiencing continuous excruciating pain in his left leg. At a loss for any other solution, his surgeon advised him to have his left leg amputated.

Not ready to agree to this, Hans was sent to Jan for physical therapy to try to stimulate re-vascularization. However, the several months of physical therapy were unsuccessful. He still had to leave his bed four times a night because of unbearable pain. He walked with two crutches and could hardly put any pressure on his foot at any time.

While working with Hans, Jan decided that the most helpful thing might be to let him talk about his situation. If he talked long enough, Jan reasoned, perhaps he would eventually make up his mind to have the needed amputation.

Then Jan learned about meridian tapping. He immediately thought of Hans. Hans resisted the idea at first, but finally gave in.

Directly following his first treatment Hans felt less stiffness in his left foot. This was enough to give him confidence in the technique. Jan gave him a setup phrase to use at home and told him to keep doing EFT, the form of meridian tapping Jan was using.

Two days later Hans returned. He had been doing his homework and reported that he now felt even more change in his left foot; there were fewer cramps, and the stiffness had begun to change. He confessed that he'd been tapping in secret because he didn't want his wife to think he also had a circulation problem in his *brain*!

After several weeks of tapping, Hans could bear more weight and stand longer on his foot and was sleeping the whole night through. With the use of tapping and the intensified exercise as the result of the changes in his legs, his condition began to improve, slowly but surely.

At present, Hans uses hardly any pain medication and is only taking 25% of the anti-coagulant medicine he needed before. He is able to work in his garden if he sits down and rests once in a while. He only uses his crutches when he walks long distances. He tells Jan that he can play some football with friends by "shooting the ball to one another." Measurements of his circulation show definite improvement. His surgeon is astonished and no longer recommends amputation. Jan has not told the surgeon that he uses meridian tapping with Hans, though, because "he is a 'real man of science'" and Jan is afraid he might disapprove.

Often tapping produces One-Minute Wonders, but for very serious and challenging conditions such as this it may need to be applied for weeks, months or even years. Still, if it can produce benefits such as Hans is experiencing, isn't it worth the relatively minor effort it requires?

Short Takes

We could fill several books with inspiring stories of pain relief through tapping. Here are just a few short takes:

A "Cool" New Move

Angela Seaman writes:

My 8-year-old-son Joseph was bouncing on my bed showing me some "cool new moves" when all of a sudden he fell onto the bed and twisted his foot. He immediately began to cry. I looked at his foot and there was a large bump a couple of inches up from his big toe. His toe was swollen as was the area around his ankle.

When I asked him to move his foot, he was unable to do so without a lot of pain and tears. I immediately began to tap on him. Amazingly enough, after each round, the swelling in all areas of his foot had gone down!!! After approximately 6-7 rounds, the bump was barely visible, there was no other swelling, and he was able to walk on the foot again!

An 84-Year Wonder

One day Allan Kreust noticed an 84-year-old neighbor with her right arm in a sling. She had pulled her shoulder out of the socket by moving a heavy suitcase. Her doctor informed her that she had damaged her muscles and ligaments. She would require at least six months of healing and might never regain full use of the arm.

Allan offered meridian tapping. "On starting, she said the 1-10 level of intensity of the pain was a 20. The first round brought it down to an 8. She was flabbergasted."

After the second round of tapping, "she removed the sling, and whirled her arms about. Needless to say, I was then the one that was flabbergasted." And how is she doing now? "She has not had a pain since and uses her arm as she always has."

From Ten to Zero — A Finger Injury

Debra Albert is a self-described "EFT Newcomer" who had powerful results. In her own words:

Earlier this summer I was doing some gardening and pinched my finger on the blade between the handles of my garden shears. The entire end of my ring finger... became purple as blood pooled under the skin. The pain was at least a 10. In fact, I was fighting to keep from passing out. I was alone at the time and managed to get inside and ice the finger but found I had to lie down. The pain was so bad that I was still on the verge of fainting. Suddenly I remembered EFT! I began to tap. *Even though I have really hurt my finger... Even though I feel like I am going to pass out... Even though I am really scared...*

After about 6 or 7 rounds all that was left was a small dot of blood on the pad of my finger tip. The pain was completely gone and my finger was not even sore.

A Few Quick Tips

When it comes to pain, tapping works for each of us in different ways, at different speeds and at different levels of permanency. For some it does not work at all, although the majority who try it do experience noticeable relief.

Here are a few mental approaches you might want to try as you experiment to find the ways that tapping works best for you.

Reframe the Pain — This technique involves thinking of the pain as *evidence of healing*, rather than as physical distress. As the body repairs itself, we often feel some measure of pain, itching, burning and other types of discomfort. Reframing the pain means simply to regard it as the body repairing itself. When we tap using statements that reframe the pain as a signal of healing, we can often notice dramatic shifts after just a few rounds. Emotional pain can be approached in this way too. (See detailed discussion of this topic in my book, *Multiply the Power of EFT*.)

Focus Away From the Pain — Anyone who has spent time with children knows that it's often easy to get a child to forget about an injury just by engaging her mind in something else. Adults are no different — take our minds off the pain and the pain goes away.

The principle is simple. Whatever we focus our attention on increases. An easy way to refocus pain is to mentally scan the body to find an area that *does* feel comfortable. Then tap using tapping statements to shift your focus to that body area. Focusing on a body part that feels pleasant is a ready tool for lessening pain.

Stop Fighting the Pain — A large part of physical pain and discomfort stems from our *resistance* to it. We think the pain shouldn't be there or is "wrong," so we fight it mentally and emotionally, which actually turns the pain meter way up. The simple act of accepting the pain (with or without using tapping) often brings it down many steps on the pain meter.

You can take this a step further by actually sending *loving attention* to the pain. By "entering into" the pain lovingly and fearlessly, rather than running away from it, the pain often melts away or turns into a feeling that's less "negative." Try using tapping statements such as *"Even though I have this pain I choose to give it loving attention,"* or, *"Even though I have this pain I choose to hear its cry, and give it love."* When pain is seen as a friend in need, not an enemy, the entire healing process can be accelerated.

In the next chapter we will look briefly at many other uses of tapping. Some of these may surprise you!

Tapping "Choices" for Pain, Illness or Injury

Even though I have this (*pain, illness, injury etc.*)...

...I choose to *flow with* the pain (*illness, injury etc.*).

...I choose to let go of my anger at the pain (*illness, injury etc.*).

...I choose to let go of struggling against the pain (*illness, injury etc.*).

...I choose to make peace with this pain (*illness, injury etc.*).

...I choose to find an unexpected strength in myself at this time.

...I choose to enjoy the things I *can* do.

...I choose to feel confident that my body can heal itself.

...I choose to heal surprisingly quickly.

I consider tapping the "people's method". It is there for all of us... literally at our fingertips.*

Dr. Patricia Carrington
Ph.D., EFT Master, EFT Cert-Honors
Founder of the Choices Tapping Method

Tapping is an ever present help in trouble, and it's free to every person.

*Quote from Dr. Patricia Carrington from the movie, _The Tapping Solution._

Chapter 14

Try Tapping for Just About Everything

In my opinion, meridian tapping is being radically underused. It has not reached its full potential by any means. It is still "in the closet," so to speak, leaving much pain and misery untreated that could easily be avoided.

Even if we were to follow this book's often repeated advice to "try it on everything," most of us would needlessly restrict its uses due to limitations in our own imagination.

We are somewhat like the computer newbie who buys a top-of-the-line machine because he's heard it's "the best" and wants nothing less for himself and his family. This computer is so powerful that it can run every application on the planet, has the maximum speed and memory currently achievable and comes equipped with all the latest high-tech features. In short, it's an electronic marvel. This thing could run NASA!

The novice owner rushes home with his new purchase, tears excitedly into the box and exclaims, "Great! Now I can get email from my family from all over the world and see pictures of my grandkids the day they're taken!"

Of course he is correct, this machine will do these things, but what he does not know is that such a basic purpose could just as easily be served with a much cheaper, less sophisticated models. The novice computer user simply does not have the experience and background to realize what amazing capabilities lie within this new machine. The things it can do for him in many other areas of his life may remain forever a secret because he does not think to explore the possibilities. Due to an innocent ignorance, it doesn't occur to him.

This is like buying a Mercedes to do the weekly grocery shopping, but never taking it on the highways.

That's the way most people use meridian tapping. It serves them for a limited purpose, for which they are grateful, but they never "take it out on the highway." I'd like to encourage you to *really* try it on *everything*: relationship problems, money concerns, allergies, "bad luck," workplace conflicts, motivational issues, goals, problems with your pet, bad habits... the list is endless.

If you're stuck in any area of your life, *try tapping*; it's that simple.

Tapping doesn't work on every issue for every person as I have said, but what is the harm in trying it? If you don't "try it on everything" you'll never unlock all of its powers. You will keep them a box. You'll be using your new state-of-the-art computer to email family photos.

In this chapter we'll look at just a few of the many, many uses that are being revealed, every day for meridian tapping. I wouldn't be surprised if the next amazing application is the one that you yourself discover!

Using Tapping to Create Desirable Habits

By far the most common use of tapping is to handle problems and roadblocks in life, but it can also be remarkably effective in helping you rid yourself of behaviors that are not serving you — undesirable habits. The only real way to change self-defeating habits is to replace them with self-enhancing ones. Meridian tapping is a powerful tool to help you do just that.

Here's an example from my practice. My client "Emily" had avoided addressing a certain frustrating habit of hers because she considered it too trivial to waste therapy sessions on. One day, however, she spontaneously mentioned that she was "sick and tired" of misplacing her numerous pairs of reading glasses and repeatedly having to buy replacements.

As someone who has lost her share of reading glasses, I sympathized and asked, "Would you like to use tapping to take away your tendency to misplace your glasses?"

"What an idea!" she said, and agreed enthusiastically.

As we explored some new solutions for keeping track of her glasses, one obvious idea came up — to create designated "parking places" and never put the glasses anywhere but in those spots. Emily knew this would be a good solution — she thought of it herself — but she was quick to add that she didn't like it. The idea would work "if only I would do it, but of course I won't."

I then asked her a pointed question, "What would be the downside to this plan?" In other words, what would she find unpleasant about implementing her own solution?

She answered immediately, "It would make me feel imposed upon. I'd resent being forced to put my glasses in a particular spot. When I'm in my own house I want to feel free!"

Emily had hit upon an important reason why many people refuse to change their behavior even when changing it would clearly be to their own advantage. Nobody likes to feel *forced* to do something — even if it's for their own good. When we do this we end up creating an inner dialogue that's more like a teacher scolding a student than a respectful, peer-to-peer adult exchange. If we adopt this kind of attitude it's bound to create inner rebellion.

So we went to work on changing her approach. She started with the tapping statement, "Even though I don't want to be forced to put my glasses in any one spot, I choose to be flexible and understanding with myself about this." Using this statement shifted her attitude and she was now ready to take it to the next step. "Even though it's a bother to walk over and put my glasses in a certain spot each time, I choose to find it interesting and satisfying to do this."

Emily had uncovered a second important truth about changing habits. *Until we can create or discover something positive and pleasurable in the new habit, we're never going to adopt it.* After our tapping session, Emily began deliberately to take pleasure in the neatness and accuracy with which she could place her glasses in the new spot. It was just a tiny thing — the placing of the glasses — but enough to give the action a positive feeling that outweighed any sense of burden.

You can use this same simple two-step process to help with any behavior you might want to change: 1) Look for the downside of changing your habit and address this with tapping. For example, replace self-imposed coercion with understanding and encouragement. Then, 2) seek something distinctly *pleasant* in the new behavior and use tapping to install a positive attitude toward your new plan. When you do this, be prepared to watch old habits melt away and new ones bloom.

Tapping Directly on Emotional States

I have talked about using tapping to work on emotions that *underlie* pains, fears, overeating and other issues, but can tapping be used *directly* on emotional states that we want to change? The answer is yes, absolutely. Tapping has brought about remarkable changes for many people who have been locked in persistent guilt, sadness, hatred, anger, resentment and other joy-stifling emotions, often for years.

Depression. Some practitioners are even reporting great success in using tapping for debilitating mood disorders such as depression. As a psychologist, I am reluctant to use tapping as the *sole* treatment for serious depression however, although I use it by itself with some mild or transient depressions. I will typically ask a *seriously* depressed client to use medication *along with meridian tapping* until such time as they are feeling substantially better. The dual use of anti-depressive medication and tapping can often facilitate the tapping process so markedly that the client can eventually taper off of the medication and rely on tapping alone. Meridian tapping can make a wonderful adjunct to other forms of therapy, when the person and therapist are ready to use it in this fashion.

Anger and Hatred. The following story reported by meridian tapping experts Philip and Jane Mountrose illustrates how intense hatred can be cleared up through the use of tapping. Philip teaches in a group home for severely emotionally disturbed teenaged boys. Not surprisingly, one of the main problems the boys have had in the mainstream school system is getting along peacefully with others. Typically, these young men bear a lot of hatred and anger.

One particular student, "Jerome," came to the group home following an arrest for drug abuse and other criminal behavior. He immediately had a hard time fitting in because of his strong feeling that his fellow residents were unforgivable, even though their offenses were in many cases no worse than his own.

Jerome's hatred toward the others was so severe that he was essentially non-functional. He preferred remaining isolated all day in the "time-out" area than to participate in any classes and activities with the others, whom he judged inferior to him. He lobbied to be removed from the group home, even if it meant returning to the far less pleasant environs of juvenile hall.

Philip decided to take a walk with Jerome and see if he could learn why Jerome was so judgmental. During their talk, he offered EFT and Jerome agreed.

Jerome tapped on his hatred toward the other boys, which was "unbearably high," in his own words. After a few rounds the teenager reported feeling better and Philip observed that he physically looked much more relaxed.

Jerome dutifully practiced tapping on himself over the weekend and on Monday was back in class with the others. After softball practice that afternoon, he approached Philip and reported that his intense feelings of hatred were completely gone. He expressed hope and optimism about remaining in the group home and has not had any problems of this type since (he continues to tap occasionally.)

Ann Adams, who also works with emotionally disturbed children, adds, "I have been using tapping in the form of EFT for several years to help emotionally disturbed children in our residential treatment center control socially disruptive and/ or self-destructive behavior... I have *never seen the tapping fail* to calm a child quickly even when they were under extreme stress..." Rehana Webster, who works with hardened recidivist criminals in New Zealand, concurs, stating, "My records show that after using meridian tapping, 95% of those people succeeded in making positive changes in their thinking and behavior, whereas other programs… had shown only a 20% success rate. According to these offenders, tapping is 'totally amazing' — I find that it is self-empowering, safe, simple to administer and to learn, and achieves lasting results…"

This is a powerful use of meridian tapping. One can imagine a world where even racism, religious intolerance and other forms of "institutionalized" hatred might be routinely tackled by applying it in time.

Meridian Tapping and Children

Meridian tapping is truly an amazing tool for children. A sizeable number of parents, educators, counselors and others who deal with children report highly successful results using tapping with a wide variety of children's issues. One intriguing development in this area is the use of a therapeutic tapping toy known as TappyBear. This stuffed animal is manufactured with tapping spot buttons strategically located on its head and upper torso and is a great facilitator of tapping, the children often tap on the bear or themselves with greater ease than they tap alone or with their parents. They seem to prefer to use meridian tapping for "Tappy's" problems rather than for their own, although they themselves show the beneficial results from having done so (for information on TappyBear see Resources Section).

Many people are surprised to learn that the use of tapping is not restricted to teens and adults. In fact, one of its most exciting and dramatic applications is for children's issues. Tapping is being used with remarkable success on children *from birth* up to the official end of "childhood" at age 14 for difficulties as diverse as:

- Colic
- Tantrums
- Nightmares
- Teething pain
- Restlessness
- ADHD symptoms

- Rashes
- Stage fright
- Bedwetting
- Bullying issues
- Stuttering
- Reading problems
- Separation anxiety

...and many others.

This is only a fraction of the listing I could give. Parents, grandparents, friends, teachers, babysitters, therapists and physicians are all successfully using tapping for an enormous range of children's issues. Just one example is the story about an eight-year-old boy with major fear issues reported by Joan Costello *(edited slightly)*:

> Tommy's mother is a mentally ill drug addict who has not been around most of his life. He is being raised by his grandparents. He bonded with his mother as a baby, but since then has had major issues of abandonment and feeling responsible for her wellbeing.
>
> He sees his mother once or twice a month under supervised visits. At the age of about 4, his mother's boyfriend held Tommy over the railing of a railroad bridge as a threat toward his mother. Although his grandparents had Tommy in traditional therapy, his fears relating to that incident are still there. Recently, this man came back into his mother's life, and Tommy has had nightmares, fear of being alone, fear of the dark, fear for his mom.
>
> Tommy is very open and talks about his fears with nothing held back. Unfortunately, he also does not want to be singled out as someone with a "problem," so we asked his 4-year-old cousin Jenny to join us when we tapped on being afraid of things that aren't there. We began our tapping with Jenny being afraid of her

dark closet. *"Even though the closet is very dark, I know it is just my clothes hanging there and I am safe."* I added some humor about dressing a scarecrow or snowman in our clothes, getting giggles out of them.

Then we moved on to Tommy's fears: *"Even though that man called the house last week and asked for my mom, he isn't here, and I am safe with my grandma and grandpa."* *"Even though I am afraid to be alone, my family is in the house with me and I have a lot of love protecting me."* *"Even though I am still afraid, all I have to do is walk into the next room, and I am not alone."* *"Even though that man was very bad to me when I was little, I am okay now — safe in my home."*

Tommy has had 3 sessions, and calls me when a situation triggers his fears. The difference in him is amazing. He doesn't call out in a panic when alone in a room. He isn't afraid to wait at the end of the driveway for the school bus, and his nightmares have stopped. Thank God, most children don't have to deal with issues like these.

What an amazing new tool meridian tapping gives us! We can only guess what will transpire when it becomes more widely known by parents, educators and others — it could well help to create a new generation of children who will have happier and healthier childhoods and, because of this, can eventually contribute to the world in new and exciting ways.

Tapping and... *Animals*?!

You definitely do not need to be human to experience the benefits of tapping. One of the most stunningly successful uses of tapping is with animals. In the same way that many animals have responded beautifully to acupuncture, thousands of dogs, cats, horses and other creatures have benefited from having their owners, trainers, veterinarians or other human friends use tapping for their behavior problems and physical distress.

In some instances people tap directly on the animals, in other cases they use surrogate or proxy tapping — tapping on themselves while using (or thinking) the animal's name. Both approaches seem to be equally effective — it seems to be the belief system and comfort level of the person (or the circumstances of the problem) that determines which approach is chosen. The effects of using meridian tapping on animals, whichever way it is applied, are often immediate and dramatic.

Although tapping does not always work on animals, because it is so highly effective when it does, and is such a gentle and noninvasive technique, it would seem well worth trying in any case of animal distress. I have used it many, many times with my own pets and only once has it failed to work.

The following story *(slightly edited)*, reported by Marina Bagley, is typical of the sudden and inexplicable results often seen with animal use.

> I recently had a great success with my mother's 10-year-old dog Snowy. She was absolutely terrified of fireworks and would shiver and shake for hours and run away in a crazy panic if she could get out of the house! Fireworks have been a nightmare for my mother for years because of her dog's problem... until now.
>
> I tapped on the dog a week ago over the Christmas break because we were in the country and the family was clay-bird shooting with a shotgun. The noise wasn't too bad but Snowy began her usual antics and managed to escape and ran down the highway for miles before we could retrieve her.
>
> After we brought her back she was so stressed with the continuing banging noise from the shotgun that she knocked my 80-year-old Mum over trying to run away again. Mum and my sister were both holding onto her and trying to calm her down and I thought, "Oh what's to lose? Even if everyone thinks I'm crazy, I'll try tapping." Even though I had no idea how to tap on an animal!

So, tapping gently on the top of head and around the chest area, I began. I worked my way down to her doggy toes and tapped on the edge of her nails, as we do on the fingernail points (using the Long Form of EFT) then back to the head. I was saying in my mind, "Even though I'm afraid of that noise, etc., and continued for some time.

She calmed right down and was no longer even reacting to the shots going off outside. Mum was surprised but very convinced that something had indeed worked. Then a week later on New Year's Eve we had a chance to test out the effectiveness of the tapping when fireworks started going off.

Snowy rushed over to sit next to Mum. Mum tapped her on the head as I had done and after a while Snowy went off by herself, lay down, and took a nap, completely unfazed by the fireworks. This was totally abnormal for her and everyone in the family was amazed.

No one can say, "It's all in the dog's mind," can they?

The sensitivity and creativity with which pet owners and others have applied this method to their animals' problems is admirable. I am enormously impressed by the potential of EFT (the form of meridian tapping Marina was using) in this area and would like to see it used worldwide with animals both domestic and wild. There is no telling how much suffering this could avert for both for the animals and their caring humans.

Using Tapping to "Manifest Our Dreams"

One of the most exciting uses of tapping lies in the domain of life often thought of as the "spiritual" realm. As you probably know, books such as *The Secret* and those by bestselling authors such as Wayne Dyer and Deepak Chopra have fueled a popular interest in using inner mechanisms, such as visualization and intention, to influence outer reality. I am often asked if meridian tapping ties in to this metaphysical trend. Can tapping be used to help manifest real, physical happenings in the outer world? In effect, can it help change reality itself?

I can only say that I have seen tapping produce some extremely promising results in this area, though I must offer a caution as well, which I'll explain in a few moments.

Let's first consider how something as immaterial as meridian tapping could possibly affect the world outside our own minds. We could fill several books with an attempt to answer that question, even though science has as yet barely broken ground in this exciting new frontier. But let's just remember, for now, that energy systems are not restricted to the dimensions of the human body. We have already noted that the electric fields generated by the heart, for example, extend well beyond the body's outer skin. We have also seen that techniques such as surrogate-tapping and animal-tapping *work*, even though classical physics would be at a loss to explain just how this happens.

As quantum physics points out, however, everything is ultimately energy and energy fields are inextricably intertwined with one another. Even matter itself is just another form of energy.

Spiritual masters and theoretical physicists are finally concurring that beneath the surface of reality, where things appear to be separate, there is a fundamental level of existence at which everything is unified. Everything really is one; we just don't see it that way with our everyday senses.

So… if (1) everything is energy and (2) everything is connected, then it is no great leap to see how a change within my own energy system or yours might affect the world at large. But beyond this, let's not continue with speculation. My suggestion is to try meridian tapping on any goal you might have, inner *or* outer, and see what happens for you. Become a pioneer. That's what "Pete," a former client of mine, did.

Pete is an experienced "Tapper" who has taken my Choices Method in a new direction. Instead of using the phrase, "*I choose to…*" in his tapping statements, he uses the phrase, "*I thank the universe for…*"

Pete's car, for example, had seen better days. He wanted a

new one but could not imagine any logical way in which he could find and afford the one he wanted. He had searched the internet for months, to no avail. It finally dawned on him to try tapping, and he formulated the following statement, *"Even though I don't know how this can happen, I thank the universe for giving me a light blue Model 240 Volvo station wagon made in the years '91 to '93."*

Note the specificity he used in his statement — that's a key part of this story. Pete tapped on this statement for a couple of weeks, then, lo and behold, an ad appeared in an online forum, offering a "Light blue 1992 Model 240 Volvo wagon" for sale. It was exactly the car Pete wanted, but the question still remained: how would he pay for it? Because it was such an old car, no banks would offer financing. He tapped for this issue, too.

As it happened, Pete had been managing some property for a bank executive who liked his work. Pete asked the man about a loan and the executive was quickly able to arrange one through his bank at the lowest possible interest rates. Pete is certain that his tapping was the key to manifesting the results he was seeking in all their wonderful detail.

Here's the important caveat that I mentioned about using tapping for manifesting. Some time later, Pete was contemplating a career change, and he decided to use meridian tapping to bring an excellent job offer. However, in this instance he found that he had difficulty formulating the right tapping statements. As he explored this problem in therapy he came to realize that he was actually conflicted about the job. Even though it would be an excellent opportunity to get that kind of job, it would also entail some lifestyle changes about which he was clearly ambivalent — he might jeopardize his current relationship by having to work in another city, for example. Pete knew that he had to work on the inner conflict before he could produce successful outer results. (How can the universe help us, after all, if it doesn't even know clearly what we want?!)

It's important, when tapping for positive life changes, that we are completely *congruent* with regard to the change. Manifesting a car was relatively simple for Pete because all parts of him were on board, he wanted the car with "his whole heart." There were no inner conflicts. But he did not want the job with "his whole heart," in fact, he was quite conflicted about it.

Often there are parts of you that want a change while other parts do not. In these cases, you must ask yourself what you *really* want. Only then does it make sense to use tapping to help bring that goal to you.

My sense is that for the majority of major life changes, even the very positive ones, some inner conflict is usually present. What will you have to give up in order to achieve your goal? What is the downside of success? Is there a "little voice inside" crying out in protest against reaching it?

The good news is that we can use tapping to root out and explore these hidden conflicts. Sometimes our inner objections can be removed. Sometimes the goal itself needs adjusting. As we get clearer on what we really want and are able to put fears and outdated emotions to rest, we are better able to move forward with truly positive goals and to manifest our dreams.

Even More Avenues for Using Meridian Tapping

Again, I want to emphasize my belief that "the sky's the limit" when it comes to using meridian tapping. Here are just a few more areas to consider. It is by no means a complete list.

Sleep Issues. Almost everyone experiences occasional problems with sleep, and some people find it extremely difficult to fall asleep, night after night. Tapping can help in both cases.

When dealing with sleep issues, it is usually helpful to use "mental tapping." That is, you don't physically tap on your body but tap only in the imagination.

Sleep can't be forced, but only "allowed." Therefore it is also often helpful to use tapping statements that do not refer *directly* to the act of falling asleep, but just encourage you to feel "pleasantly drowsy." Once in this state, sleep usually follows naturally. If some worry is preventing you from falling asleep, use a tapping statement that directs your subconscious to work out that issue while you peacefully sleep.

Addictions. In the proper hands, meridian tapping has been used to combat some major addictions with surprising success. This usually occurs over a period of time, however, as these conditions require persistence.

Because addictive behavior is complex, the person caught in it usually needs support and guidance as they work their way through the maze of deeply troubling issues involved. Meridian tapping's long-term successes in the area of addictions are due to its ability to address the true cause of most addictions, namely the need to "tranquilize" the anxiety that stems from one's underlying anger, fear, guilt, trauma, etc. We looked at this dynamic in the chapter on weight loss.

If you want to try tapping for a serious addictive problem, you may want to consider working with an experienced meridian tapping practitioner. On the other hand you may be able to clear up "minor" compulsions and cravings, using tapping on your own.

Allergies. Western medicine tends to view allergies as being chemically caused, even though the evidence for this is often weak or absent. As a result, the "cures" it offers typically come from a pharmacy.

True cures, however, rarely result from taking medications. All we usually get from meds is partial symptom relief. Tapping, on the other hand, tackles allergies at their root by going to work on both the body's energy system *and* the emotional conditions that frequently underlie allergies. People all over the world have reported using tapping to produce "miraculous" elimination of adverse reactions from hay fever, rashes, insect stings, anaphylactic shock, allergies to milk, foods, chemicals and a wide variety of environmental triggers.

Caution, of course, should be employed here, because some allergic reactions can be life threatening, but tapping often does what pharmaceuticals cannot — it can eliminate the allergy permanently.

Changing Perspective. I find that even experienced tapping users often fail to use tapping to influence the way they view their life. This is probably because most of us have trouble seeing the forest for the trees. We can recognize the details of our lives and know how to respond to them, but can be quite unaware of our underlying assumptions about life. Yet these assumptions can be running our lives.

How do you use tapping to "get at" your assumptions? One way to do this is to become aware of any hidden resistance to developing new attitudes. If you notice that you fear changing an unproductive attitude, or despair of ever being able to change it, you can begin to tap *on this resistance*. As you do this, you will often uncover assumptions and beliefs of which you have not been consciously aware. And then you can use tapping to install more positive and productive beliefs in their place.

Creating Gratitude and Appreciation.   Many spiritual traditions, both ancient and modern, stress the importance of developing a sense of gratitude in life. For many of us, however, this turns out to be more easily said than done.

This may be due to evolutionary hard-wiring. As a matter of survival, *homo sapiens* has been conditioned, as a species, to be more alert to difficulties and dangers than to conditions that are safe and working out just fine. In the wild, the sound of a cracking twig is much more attention-worthy than the sound of a peacefully babbling brook.

Meridian tapping offers a concrete way to "tap in" (install) a sense of gratitude so that it becomes a more permanent part of your life. One way to do this is to notice those things in life that give you a *genuine* sense of gratitude (not the standard list of things that *should* make you feel grateful). Perhaps you have a window that looks out on a pond and every time you gaze out of it, you get a thrill. Perhaps your work brings you intense joy and satisfaction. Once you identify that genuine feeling — including the physical sensations it produces — you can use meridian tapping to increase it.

An equally effective approach is to look for the positive moment in a negative experience and to tap on that. *"Even though I'm disappointed at the way I felt at the party yesterday, I'm grateful that I chose not to drink (or eat) too much."* Often by identifying one small positive *Aspect*, other positive memories start to flow and what had previously seemed to be a negative experience turns into something much richer. Using tapping in this way can retrain the mind to focus on gratitude much more often and much more automatically.

Think about what issues you are struggling with in your life. Low self-esteem? Relationship problems? Lack of purpose? Loneliness? Boredom? Another? Then try tapping to open an inner dialogue with yourself and start the process of change. The good thing is that you can start exactly where you are at this moment. Tapping will then lead you to the next door that needs to be opened, and then the next...

Only the future will tell what limitations, if any, there are to this remarkable new energy method called meridian tapping. We will explore what that future may hold in our last chapter.

Tapping "Choices" for Anger

Even though I feel angry (*furious, enraged etc.*) at (*fill in the person or situation that is angering you*)...
...I choose to keep a level head about this.
... I choose to use my anger to strengthen me.
... I choose to use my anger appropriately and well.
... I choose to find a solution that will be helpful to everyone concerned.

Tapping "Choices" for Sadness

Even though I feel sad (depressed etc.)...
... I choose to remember how much support I have from others (*if this rings true*).
... I choose to know that this sadness too will pass.
... I choose to notice *good* feelings I had today.

Part 4

The Meridian Tapping Retreat

If someone can be traumatized in thirty seconds, why can't they be healed in a day, an hour, a minute?*

Rick Wilkes
Founder of "Thriving Now"
Meridian Tapping Expert

Tapping brings about healing through intervention in the human energy system, one of the reasons for its amazing rapidity.

*Quote from Rick Wilkes in the movie, *The Tapping Solution.*

Chapter 15

Overview

On October 26, 2007, ten people who were strangers to each other assembled from various parts of the United States and Canada at the Clear Point Center in Stafford Springs, Connecticut. They were there to embark on a four-day adventure into what they had been told was an exciting new energy healing method called meridian tapping. The one thing these ten people had in common was desperation. They had tried many methods to help with their problems, but nothing had worked. For most of them, meridian tapping was their last hope.

Cameras would be running 24 / 7 throughout their stay and all ten knew and accepted that. They also knew that intensely personal, even painful, details about their lives would be captured on video, perhaps to be shared with the world. They were willing to pay that price. They had come to Clear Point ready to change.

By the end of the four-day workshop those ten strangers would feel like family. Many of them would have experienced life-changing experiences, real turning points. And *we* would be the beneficiaries of their courage and openness, thanks to the film of that extraordinary event known as *The Tapping Solution*.

The workshop was the brainchild of creator-producer Nick Ortner. He didn't want the film to be merely informational and inspirational or to paint an unrealistic picture, seen through rose-colored glasses. He wanted to show tapping *in action*, with real people and real life problems. He wanted to capture the successes, the failures, the joys, the struggles.

The ten participants were chosen from among more than one hundred and fifty applicants. Each had filled out a preliminary application form and participated in exploratory interviews. Though some degree of subjective intuition was used, the main criteria for acceptance were: the applicants' willingness to try tapping; their willingness to continue doing it after the event; their diversity in terms of age, race, gender, income level, etc.; and the likelihood that a general audience could relate to their problems. Only one of the chosen applicants had dabbled in tapping before; most had not tried it. The organizers – Nick, his sister Jessica Ortner, and colleague Nick Polizzi, the main cameraman and film editor – were looking for a broad spectrum of people and life issues. Some of the applications just seemed to "glow" or stand out in some way.

Clear Point was a perfect setting to hold and film the event – woods, hiking trails, natural foods were all a part of it. All ten participants were required to stay on site for the full four days (except for one participant who had to leave briefly to receive methadone treatment on a set schedule). They shared bedrooms, dined together and spent their leisure time together.

The workshop days consisted of two main activities: (1) learning about and doing meridian tapping together as a group (focusing on one individual at a time as the rest of the group tapped along), and (2) doing private one-on-one tapping sessions with trained practitioners. Cameras were always on, in both the group room and the "private" room. A third room was available in which no cameras were present. This room was for needed moments of complete privacy and for off-camera sessions, which were sometimes done as part of the process.

Besides Nick Ortner, the meridian tapping experts who ran the program and conducted the individual sessions were Helena Johnson, Steve Munn and Rick Wilkes. Steve runs Clear Point and had generously offered its use for the retreat. Jessica Ortner provided the weekly coaching by phone that was offered to all of the participants as a follow-up to the live workshop. Not surprisingly, those participants who took advantage of the weekly coaching sessions were generally those who reported the strongest long-term results.

In the following pages we will take a brief look at each of the ten participants, in a Before, During and After format. We will discover why they volunteered for the program in the first place, what went on for them during the workshop and how they are doing now, six months later. The three facilitators, Steve, Rick and Helena, and visiting meridian tapping expert Carol Look (who spent the last day with the participants) contributed their valuable insights to this section of the book. If you haven't yet seen the film, *The Tapping Solution,* formerly known as *Try It On Everything,* I would recommend you watch it before reading this section. It is not entirely necessary of course, but the following material does "give away" certain happenings in the film and is better appreciated against the backdrop of the film.

Now let's visit our ten participants. We will meet them in alphabetical order since no one person is more important than another in this universal drama...

Chapter 16

Bernadette's Story

Before

On the application form for the four-day tapping workshop, question number eight read, "On a scale of one to ten, how much of a role does stress play in your life?" Bernadette's answer was, "Ten."

As a single working mother who had raised four sons on her own, it's easy to see why. Although her sons are now adults, Bernadette's answers to the other questions on the application form reveal a greater and more immediate stressor in her life: a recent diagnosis of blocked arteries, high cholesterol, pre-hypertension, and pre-diabetes. During the admission process, Bernadette reported that she had been steadily gaining weight for twenty years. She feared that her combination of poor eating habits and thickening artery walls rendered her, "a heart attack in the making." To add further urgency to the matter, she was due to lose her health insurance in a matter of months.

A perfect storm was taking shape in her life.

For years Bernadette had struggled with food issues. For instance, she loved Dunkin Donuts. Every time she passed one of the shops, an internal tug-of-war would begin: "Do I buy a donut or not?" If she saw a dessert table filled with cakes and pastries, she would vividly imagine eating all of the sweets. This idea triggered intense emotional warfare. Should she eat the food and enjoy the emotional balm it offered or make the healthy choice? This type of battle consumed a lot of her inner energy.

The good news was, Bernadette seemed to have much to live

for and wanted to be free from her struggles. On her application she described herself as "very engaged" with family and friends, and reported a rich and vital spiritual life. She seemed to have many positive motivations for living a long, healthy life and was very open to trying new therapies.

Bernadette had, in fact, already sampled meridian tapping. Prior to the heart catheterization procedure that diagnosed her blocked arteries, she was given a session of tapping by a meridian tapping practitioner and it had helped her relax. She'd retained an interest in the method and had always intended to learn more about it.

Looking back on herself prior to the workshop, Bernadette now says, "I feel like I had some issues *stuck in my cells*." These seemed to be engrained issues that mentally-oriented treatments could not address. That was what interested her in the body-energy approach that meridian tapping represented.

During

Bernadette arrived at the workshop late. She seemed ready to work, but perhaps a bit more guarded and reserved than most of the others. She was the only participant, for instance, who did not want to share photos of her family. She clearly had a "sweet heart," says Helena, "but didn't seem to have a strong desire to open up".

Helena decided that it would be best to work with Bernadette privately, off-camera, before asking her to work in front of the group. Trust quickly developed between the two women and Bernadette revealed that during her difficult years of being a single, working mother to four sons, she had come to view lunchtime as the highlight of her day. It was her only time to be alone and to enjoy pure and simple pleasure. Food had consequently taken on a high emotional value for her.

As they tapped, Bernadette went back in time, in her imagination, to a moment when she clearly remembered feeling very excited about food. Helena asked her to reframe this excitement in a new way, encouraging Bernadette to consider the idea that her excitement about mealtime wasn't necessarily about the food itself, but was about the idea of having time to herself, time to reflect and relax. Bernadette discovered that, as a busy mom and professional counselor, she had come to feel that her life had no purpose for herself, only for others. With some tapping, she began actually to feel good about herself.

At a later point, when working in front of the group, Bernadette was given a large chocolate chip cookie that she really wanted to eat "right now." She tapped about the craving, then afterwards tasted the cookie and found it didn't taste as good as she thought it would. When it was suggested to her that she share the large cookie with the rest of the group, her face dropped – she did not want to do it. They tapped about sharing the cookie, then afterwards Bernadette found she actually *wanted* to share. She gave most of the cookie away, keeping only a small piece for herself.

The theme of this exercise, and many of the others that Bernadette was led through during the four-day retreat, was to help Bernadette feel comfortable *with or without the* food, as long as she felt happy and comfortable with herself.

After

Bernadette's story since the workshop has been one of steady growth and positive progress although not necessarily dramatic success. She is a bit disappointed that she has not lost the weight she hoped she would lose. When asked about her relationship with food since attending the program, she describes it as definitely changing but not completely changed.

Yet some of her other comments suggest that her life changes have been more sweeping. For example, she now reports that she is no longer angry at herself for being overweight. She is more relaxed in her approach to weight loss and doesn't beat herself up so much anymore. She has already lost seven pounds. She has not given up the *intention* to continue to lose weight, but she has given up the constant sense of *struggle*.

"I no longer feel food is controlling me," she says. For example, she reports that she can now walk into a Dunkin Donuts and order coffee without even thinking about buying a donut.

She often doesn't realize, until later, that the purchase took place without the familiar inner struggle over the donut – it just wasn't an issue.

Whenever she has cravings or "negative emotions about food," she says she taps about it and is able to regain equanimity.

Bernadette also taps on an as-needed basis to help her deal with stress. "I use tapping as a tool when I recognize I'm in a distressed state and I don't want to be there. I know that I can tap on that emotion and work with it. When I do that, I can always reduce my stress." She cites as an example a recent stressful period when she was starting a new job. She would make regular trips to the ladies' room, tap for a few minutes, then return to work in a more peaceful frame of mind. "It was really helpful," she says.

Bernadette clearly sees the benefit of tapping and acknowledges that she does not use the technique as often as she thinks would be desirable. She says she taps perhaps once a day, five days a week, but often only for a few minutes. When she does tap, she usually focuses on relieving her stress without taking the time to really focus on her challenges. She now believes that being more consistent and really taking the time to search for the root of her problem would give her more benefits. This is likely true. (See the book, *Multiply the Power of EFT*, listed in the Resources Section, for information on ingenious ways to build tapping into your daily routine.)

For those considering tapping, Bernadette suggests, "Try it. You have nothing to lose. It's easy, simple, and it works. Anybody can do it and it doesn't take long to learn." She heartily endorses tapping with a partner, because of the structure and support it offers.

"Just be open!" she cheerfully advises to anyone on the fence. She strongly intends to keep on tapping.

Bernadette's Progress

Before:

- Felt an incredible sense of stress in her life.
- Was angry and frustrated at herself about her weight. "I always beat myself up when I look in the mirror."
- Often felt "out of control" around food.
- Could not motivate herself to exercise consistently.
- Found it difficult to walk a long distance without tiring
- Was steadily gaining weight.
- Could not lose weight even when she dieted.
- Had trouble sleeping through the night because of stress.

After

- Feels less stressed.
- "I no longer beat myself up. I take everything one step at a time."
- "I feel like I have a different relationship with food. It doesn't control my life."
- Consistently walks every day for an average of 30 minutes.
- No longer gaining weight.
- Lost 7 pounds.
- No longer has trouble sleeping.
- "My relationship with my family has improved since I started using meridian tapping."
- "I feel more connected with my emotions. I can now recognize when I'm hungry or when I want to eat for emotions and then I can tap."
- Feels more balanced.

Chapter 17

Dennis's Story

Before

Dennis's application form for the tapping retreat has a noticeably different appearance from the other applications. Whereas most of his fellow participants wrote somewhat lengthy answers, often several pages, Dennis's answers are all extremely brief. The most detailed answer on his form was, "I have smoked cigarettes for 33 years and I am having a real hard time quitting. Tried numerous times with no success."

However, Dennis is not a man lacking in insight. He is a deeply spiritual man who is writing a book and trying to live the American Dream – traveling around the country with his wife, selling nutritional health products. At least one fellow retreat participant describes him as someone who had clearly "done a lot of self work." His contagious, smart sense of humor was apparent from the start of the workshop.

His brief answers seem to reflect his narrow focus. Dennis seemed to be coming to the workshop for one reason and one reason only: "Quit smoking forever!!!!" As for his *reasons* for wanting to quit, it is interesting to note that, in the very few words he chose to write on paper, these two reasons came up: "My wife hates it," and, "I am not the example I want to be to *others*." As clinicians know, when a client undertakes to stop an addiction for the sake of others, this is not a valid motivation. It almost always backfires.

During

Although Dennis came to the workshop ostensibly to quit smoking, in the end he did not quit smoking. So was Dennis a failure? Well, his story brings up a couple of fascinating questions in the world of meridian tapping. That is, can tapping help us change something that in our "heart of hearts" we don't want to change? And is failure to make a specific change necessarily a Failure with a capital F?

In the arena of meridian tapping we sometimes see people who have successfully used the technique recommend it to others. Frequently we hear them report that they are disappointed because the technique does not work as well on their spouse/ friend/colleague/family member. Why is this?

The very short answer is that tapping is not a "forcing" (guerilla) technique. We can't use it *on*, or "sell" it *to*, people who don't genuinely want to change. It's the "you can lead a horse to water, but you can't make him drink" pattern. The fact is that tapping is not a magic bullet. The decision to change must come from within. If it does not, then true motivation for change will be lacking and the technique will energetically fall flat.

The same is often true when we use tapping to change a habit or condition we *tell ourselves* we want to change, but are internally conflicted about. In Dennis's case, no one tried to *force* tapping on him, but it did become clear within the workshop environment that he felt a good deal of external pressure to change his smoking habit. Dennis was in a health-oriented business and believed that his smoking was not congruent with his new career or the image he needed to convey. He wanted to quit as a matter of integrity, he told himself and his fellow workshop participants. (He also had encouragement from a business partner to try meridian tapping to help him make this change.)

Yet the program staff had a suspicion, right from the start, that Dennis did not come to the program *just* to quit smoking. Something else was lurking just below the surface.

Meridian tapping, as a process, tends to bring out the truth. As we tap on various *Aspects* of an issue, we begin to get a clearer picture of where the real energy blocks are. What quickly emerged for Dennis as he tapped was the realization that he had always "done as he was told." He'd done things in his life because he was "supposed to" do them or because others wanted him to. A vivid illustration of this can be seen in the film when he talks about his childhood experiences of raising his hand in class when he needed to use the bathroom. One could only use the bathroom when permitted, he explained. And if the teacher didn't acknowledge your raised hand, you just had to hold it. Dennis described an incident in which he actually wet his pants in class because he could not get permission to go to the bathroom. This incident has been repeated, symbolically, in many ways in his life.

During the workshop Dennis revealed this longstanding tendency to subordinate his own needs and desires to "the rules" and the wishes of others. As he tapped on this, he came to see that his reasons for wanting to quit smoking were really for others, not for himself. He himself, in fact, got a tremendous amount of pleasure from smoking. He had never allowed himself to fully experience that pleasure, however, because he had always known smoking was "bad" and contrary to the self-image he wanted to embody.

After

In the opinion of Rick, one of the program facilitators, what Dennis accomplished via the workshop was to become, for the first time in his life, a "happy smoker." It may seem odd to portray the decision to smoke as a victory of sorts, but in Dennis's case, it represented a milestone in his life. It signified that he was finally finished with making choices for other people. He was going to start making choices for himself, even if that meant continuing, at least for now, with a habit that others might judge him negatively for. This was not an act of knee-jerk rebelliousness, Rick believes. While Dennis had often played a bit of a rebel role in his life, this was not a case of "I'm going to smoke and you can't stop me," but a case of Dennis getting to the point where he was capable of making a real choice. Even if that meant he would be "immortalized" on film as the guy who failed to quit smoking.

Dennis was finally relaxed and comfortable making a choice for himself and this was a genuine step of growth for him.

There is a principle in meridian tapping (and most forms of mental/emotional healing) that you can't move on until you fully accept where you are now. To try to do so is the equivalent of starting a car trip to a destination spot without knowing where you're starting from. Getting there would be impossible. That is why so much emphasis is placed on the all-purpose set-up phrase, "Even though I [whatever your issue is], I deeply and completely love and accept myself." We must accept ourselves with the issue before trying to change it.

While there are certainly many excellent reasons why Dennis "should" quit smoking, it wouldn't happen for him until he fully accepted himself as a smoker. And now he has. We don't know if Dennis will decide to quit smoking in the near future, but at least he got himself to a place of genuine choice. And if he can remain there (continued tapping would greatly help with this), it is entirely possible that in a few months' or a few years' time, he will make the authentic decision that he no longer wishes to smoke. And then he will have his first real chance for success in this, rather than repeating his many previous failed attempts.

Whether Dennis quits or not, he will at least have stopped ingesting the toxins of fear and self-recrimination along with the toxins of the cigarettes.

As an after note to his tapping experience, Dennis was offered the opportunity to continue weekly tapping sessions after the workshop – not for smoking (which he did not want to tap about), but for stress relief. Dennis declined the offer. We do not know why he did but can assume that it has to do with a non-readiness factor. People heal, if they are going to do so, at their own selected time and it is always their own decision as to when that will be.

Dennis's Progress

Before:

- Smoked, but wanted to quit.
- Felt lack of integrity because he smoked and sold health products.
- Troubled by being "left out" of social situations due to smoking.
- Had a lifelong habit of doing things because others wanted him to.

After:

- Still smokes, but no longer wants to quit.
- At end of workshop, had greater self-acceptance.
- At end of workshop, had greater insight into his habit of doing things for others; less desire to do so.

Chapter 18

Donna's Story

Before

Donna is a thoughtful, intelligent woman in her forties who seemed to have a clear sense of the issues in her life that were challenging her and very definite hopes for what a new technique such as meridian tapping might offer.

Six months prior to the four-day retreat, Donna, a realtor and mother of two teens, was diagnosed with Breast Cancer and had a bilateral mastectomy. She had just completed eight chemo treatments and thirty-three rounds of radiation, the last of which took place only days before the tapping workshop. She was well aware that her form of cancer "tends to be aggressive in nature with reoccurrence typical within the first year."

Along with the cancer and its treatments came what for Donna was perhaps an even more urgent concern: chronic insomnia. "I have not slept for more than a three-hour stretch since May when my chemo started. I've actually gone four days without sleep. I wake up at least three times a night and that is with two sleeping meds plus my Lexapro. I believe my body needs a chunk of time to sleep to heal. I feel I am putting my health and recovery at risk."

"My other complaint," Donna reported, "is lack of energy. I went from being a Type-A person to a complete halt. I am trying to rebuild my body and my energy level through diet but am quickly and easily fatigued. The radiation only adds to that fatigue." Donna desperately wanted her teenaged kids to "have their 'old' mom back again. I currently feel out of control and at the mercy of the medical specialists." She added, "Less anxiety and an inner peace and confidence would be a gift too. I have retreated from my previous lifestyle and social life since the chemo started. It would be great to have the confidence and energy to 'rejoin' the world again."

A "holistic-minded" person, Donna clearly felt somewhat at odds with the aggressive Western-medicine approach to treatment she'd opted to pursue. "All these toxins and medications are very damaging physically and mentally to me although I felt it was necessary to pursue [them]." She said the combination of medications, chemo and radiation, conflicted with her holistic beliefs, but also stated, "I am grateful for both eastern and western medicines to help me conquer my cancer."

Donna had tried Reiki, acupuncture and craniosacral therapy and had begun seeing a therapist to help her manage some of the issues that were causing her anxiety, yet nothing was helping her sleep. It was her therapist, in fact, who had recommended Donna apply for the workshop.

As with many busy people who are diagnosed with serious illness, Donna reported, "The cancer has been a blessing to me in many ways. It has helped me to find a balance in my life that was lacking. It has helped me to realize what is truly important to me and to evaluate what changes I need to make in my life to help me live to my potential with a joyful soul." She describes her life before the diagnosis as one of perpetual motion. "I kept myself extremely busy from sunup to sundown to avoid facing some personal circumstances. My recent illness has helped me to reevaluate every aspect of my life."

What did Donna hope to gain if she were selected for the tapping workshop? "Sleeping would be a wonderful gift to me." She also hoped for a decrease in anxiety and an increase in energy. As for her envisioned post-workshop future, "I hope my new 'normal' is different than my old normal. I so want to be a contributing member of society again and explore new ventures and enjoy my life with a new outlook and energy." She looked forward to traveling, spending more time with friends and family, and to further deepening the spiritual connections she had made during her recent medical ordeal.

On her application form, Donna wrote, in all capital letters, "PLEASE PICK ME!" She further pleaded, "I see your workshop as a new beginning for me, a way to celebrate all that I've been through and all that I have to look forward to... I would be so grateful for the opportunity."

The workshop team decided Donna should have that opportunity. She was selected as one of the ten participants.

During

When the staff began working with Donna, it soon emerged that her life issues went deeper than the cancer itself. This was not surprising. Like several of the women in the workshop, Donna had a long pattern of putting others first, to the exclusion of herself. When asked what she wanted in life, she would give answers such as, "I want my children to be happy." She spoke often of her active role as mother and the needs of her children in a way that suggested she was right in the middle of her child-rearing years. In fact, though, her children were 16 and 18 at the time. She seemed reluctant to transition out of full-time maternal mode.

In the workshop, Donna did not seem comfortable claiming personal power and did not seem to fully "inhabit" her own body. Her voice was extremely quiet.

During the workshop she began to realize that she did not know how to put herself first, how to assert her own needs or how to give herself loving, attentive care. When asked, for instance, to imagine telling her family that she was going to take a few hours to do something nice for herself, she revealed strong inner tension about it.

Donna's tapping sessions revolved around the theme of claiming and expressing her personal power. She also worked on the issue of feeling fully like a woman in the aftermath of a double mastectomy. Donna tapped about sleep issues, too, and was able to make dramatic strides in that area both during the workshop and afterwards.

Donna slept the full night the first day of the event. She was shocked. It was the first time in four months that she was able to sleep more than three hours. She slept soundly every night at the event. "When you have insomnia, having a good night's sleep is the best gift you can ask for. Being able to sleep changes everything."

After

Donna returned home from the workshop able to sleep comfortably. This was a major goal accomplished for her.

The program staff was concerned about Donna returning to the environment where she was the identified "cancer person," however. As Rick points out, "Serious disease needs to be an ongoing energetic journey." We need to be *very* attentive to our "vibrational trends" and any new determination to put ourselves first must be reinforced over and over again. It is not a light and casual life change. There was concern that Donna, and her family/social system, would not be ready to support and maintain such a sweeping, ongoing redefinition of herself.

Unfortunately, Donna *was* re-diagnosed with cancer a few months after the workshop. The good news is, she is meeting the challenge on a different level now. "When I was re-diagnosed with cancer I didn't know how I was going to be able to make it through six more months of chemo. It was an emotional blow. Then I tapped on my fears around having cancer and the treatment. I don't feel so overwhelmed now. I used to spend so much time running to a million different healers. I kept looking for ways outside of myself to heal. Tapping has given me a tool that I can use to heal my own spirit. I learned that I have the power to help myself. I feel supported and strong. I don't need to wait for help, I can tap while I'm getting the chemo. I wish I could tell others that they don't have to feel the pressure of always being "positive." I now realize the importance of *expressing* my feelings, tapping and then letting them go. It's made an immense difference in my life."

Donna's journey is an unfolding one and we wish her all the success that she so fully deserves.

Donna's Progress

Before:

- It was common to go four nights without sleep.
- "Before when I was on chemo I would just sit outside in a vegetative state and could not do anything."
- Couldn't drive kids anywhere or attend their sporting events.
- Felt at the mercy of the medical professionals.
- Could not take time for herself without feeling extreme guilt or anxiety.
- "I didn't express myself. I kept all my feeling in. I didn't feel comfortable expressing my opinions."
- "I felt uncomfortable receiving helps from others."

After:

- "I no longer wake up in the middle of the night. I feel like I'm getting the REM sleep that I never got before."
- Has the energy to participate in activities again. "I am now fully functional. I can go to my kids' events but I give myself permission to miss a few without guilt."
- "I no longer feel at the mercy of medical professionals. I still attend my appointments but I now feel like the healing comes from within."
- Can take time for herself without feeling guilt or anxiety "I feel like it's important for me to express myself and it's something I work on everyday."
- "Now that I have tapping, this round of Chemo treatment is so different."
- Is comfortable receiving help. "I now welcome help and prayers from others."

Chapter 19

Jackie's Story

Before

Jackie's own words on her workshop application eloquently capture her life challenges prior to the tapping training retreat. "My mind is holding me back from becoming the successful businessperson that I want to be. I know I have a lot of good stuff to say to people, but I get incredibly fearful of having to speak in public, or even on a conference call. It could be something as minor as going into my manager's office to ask a question. My heart starts to beat faster and I may even break out with a rash. Intellectually I know it is ridiculous... but I can't seem to help it."

A professional realtor, Jackie enjoys real estate and really wants to help people make the right decisions, but she was clearly handicapped when it came to doing things like making follow-up calls to warm prospects. While this was "THE most important thing that needed to get done," she hated doing it because she felt as if she was "bothering" people or that they would yell at her or hang up.

On the home front, her relationship with her husband was "extremely difficult." After 17 years of marriage he seemed in many ways a stranger to her. She had a very hard time complimenting him or saying, "I love you" or "thank you" to him. "I can talk to myself forever but I just can't seem to express the emotions I want to him."

Before the workshop, Jackie described her general stress level as "about a 7," which also reflected some severe money difficulties. Sometimes she would be in her car driving and for no apparent reason would just start crying

Her greatest fear? "That I will never really 'make it.' The little voice is always saying 'Yeah, but you could never do that.' My fear is that I'll never clear this blockage that is holding me emotionally hostage."

Jackie was more than enthusiastic about the possibility of participating in the workshop, and to her delight, she was chosen as a participant. She showed up for the four-day event crackling with energy and full of smiles, just a hint of apprehension showing behind her eyes.

During

Over the course of the four-day workshop, Jackie became in the words of Rick Wilkes, "a different woman."

It seems that the main problem that prompted Jackie to apply to the meridian tapping program – her fear of public speaking – actually cleared up relatively quickly and easily. When Jackie was first asked to think about an upcoming presentation she was going to make in her real estate job, her body immediately became stiff with discomfort. She literally shook with anxiety. But after a few rounds with a fairly standard tapping phobia protocol, she had lost this intensity of feeling. Jackie stood, first, on a short stool, then on a taller chair/stool and addressed the group. By the end of the workshop, she was quite comfortably speaking to the group, volunteering to work in front of the others, and reporting no anxiety about doing this.

What was lurking just behind the fear of *public* speaking, though, was a fear of *private* speaking – that is, speaking the truth in her life and her marriage. For years, Jackie had been unable to honestly talk to her husband about what she felt was a broken relationship. She had lingering anger and resentment over a bankruptcy they'd gone through, among other issues. Jackie and her husband would sometimes go for weeks without exchanging more than a handful of words. Jackie felt the relationship was over, but she could not imagine how the details of family life would be handled if they decided to go their separate ways. It all seemed impossible.

But she continued to tap about it and to explore the various *Aspects* of speaking her mind, from many different angles and perspectives. She also worked on her perfectionism and self-criticism, as shown in the film. By the end of the workshop, her entire demeanor had changed and she seemed more relaxed and confident in general.

After

Jackie's progress since the workshop has been a textbook success story, at least as she presently reports it. One could hardly ask for a stronger testimonial to the power of meridian tapping. Beginning with what was her most immediate concern – her fear of public speaking – Jackie now reports, "In the past I was terrified of speaking in front of people, now I actually *look forward* to it." Toward that end, she has joined Toastmasters, an organization devoted to helping its members develop speaking and leadership skills. Finding actual *pleasure* in public speaking is a big difference from the terror and panic she was unable to sooth before with "rational thinking."

When it comes to speaking her own personal truth, Jackie says, "I have finally found my voice.... Now if I do have something to say, I feel comfortable saying it." This shift has been most apparent in her marriage. "In the last few weeks, I've found the words that needed to be said." she reports.

She describes a sense of "huge relief" because she and her husband have been able to speak honestly. Although they have agreed to separate, they are both much happier, she says, and are both "looking forward in a more positive way." All of the details of family and property she spent years worrying about are falling into place and "being handled."

As to her life in general, Jackie reports that, "My entire outlook has shifted." As she speaks about this by phone to Jessica, she struggles a bit to find the words to express the depth of change she has experienced. For a moment she seems to lapse into her old pattern of feeling blocked and unable to express herself in words. Then she summons up the courage and clarity to speak again. "Tapping has allowed me to take my life to the next level, where I always wanted to go," she explains.

Previously, she says, she was locked into "the known." Now she feels able to step into uncharted territory and reports, "I'm *creating* my life now."

"I can absolutely shift a mood, change it in one minute. I did it this morning," She was feeling stressed by fear and so she "tapped on it and it was gone. It changed the whole focus of my day."

Jackie believes that if people can learn to tap the moment a negative emotion strikes, then pretty soon there will be no more room for negative energy in their lives and "the sky will be the limit" as to what they can achieve.

Jackie seems determined to prove this in her own life. Not only has she affected a stunning reversal in her ability to speak truthfully and control her fears, but she also reports that she has "completely turned things around" financially.

"I can feel it in my bones, in my soul, that I am going to be successful and that I can have everything I want."

Pretty impressive words for someone who, a year ago, could barely speak her mind without breaking out in a rash.

Jackie's Progress

Before:

- Terrified of public speaking.
- Dreaded making calls to potential clients.
- Fearful of contributing during conference calls.
- Talked about joining Toastmasters for years without being able to .
- Would feel tense and uncomfortable about speaking up in a business environment.
- Felt like she didn't belong when she was in a group environment.
- Unable to express herself to her husband.
- Felt stuck in a marriage.
- Felts anxiety over the logistics of a divorce.

After:

- Looks forward to public speaking.
- Began to speak in public about meridian tapping and the Movie.
- Finally joined Toastmasters.
- Now contributes during conferences.
- Feels comfortable in a group – "I feel like I belong instead of feeling like I need to shield myself from others."
- Able to express her feelings to husband.
- Decided to separate from husband.
- No longer feels anxiety over the logistics of the divorce.
- "The vision of myself has totally changes. I feel more confidence in every area of my life."

Chapter 20

Jodi's Story

Before

Jodi is an energetic and vibrant teacher, student, healer, wife and mother of four — and a writer. She applied for the four-day tapping workshop in hopes that she could rid herself of her chronic *fibromyalgia*, a condition that causes intense pain in the joints, muscles and tendons. Jodi's pain was concentrated mainly in her knees and she reported sometimes "crawling around because I was in so much pain." She'd had the syndrome for about fifteen years and along with it the sleep problems common to its sufferers. She reported that it had been many years since she'd been able to sleep through a single night. Typically she would awaken 15-20 times.

The fibormyalgia had forced some substantial lifestyle changes on Jodi. She was reduced to living on one floor of the house and was compelled to give up the daily walks in nature that she cherished as an important part of her spiritual life.

To some, hoping to rid oneself of an "incurable" condition might seem boldly optimistic, but Jodi was no stranger to bold thinking. She was a strong believer in the Law of Attraction and had long been a follower of empowerment-oriented writers and speakers such as Jack Canfield, Deepak Chopra, Esther Hicks, Wayne Dyer and Joe Vitale.

Jodi had even once conducted her own seminar on the Law of Attraction. And yet, some things were not moving in her life as she wished they would. Although Jodi appeared happy to the outside world she was suffering inside. Her past was filled with traumatic experiences, from having seen her mother being beaten by her father to discovering her daughter was HIV positive and pregnant.   Jodi's past seemed like one traumatic event after another but she was determined to teach others that they can surpass any obstacle.   Her intentions always seemed to fall short, though, as her past continued to haunt her and affect her personal and family life.

Her other main issue, with which she hoped to get help from meridian tapping, was her struggle with her writing.   Jodi wanted to be a published author and believed she had the skills and talent to do so, but she always seemed to experience blocks. "I'd get to a certain point in writing a book, then stop."

No one could accuse Jodi of being a negative or low-energy person.   Her life-force and enthusiasm jump right out at you the moment you see her.   In fact, the workshop team had told Jodi, in her official acceptance email, that the reason she'd been chosen to participate was because of her commitment to take her life to the next level.

Everyone involved in the workshop could *feel* that commitment from the moment Jodi arrived.

During

We might describe fibromyalgia (FM) as a "mystery disease." Its causes and chemistry are not fully known.   But Rick Wilkes noticed that her intense pain often seemed to be precipitated by a traumatic event, so when he first began to tap with Jodi, he explored that avenue.   He asked her if anything significant had happened in her life prior to the onset of FM.   Immediately Jodi replied that at that time she had just learned that her daughter, who'd long battled addiction, was both pregnant and HIV-positive.   When asked to describe how she felt about this, her only reply was a simple and very convincing "sad."

She moved on to speaking about the resulting knee pain from the fibromyalgia that had forced her to give up her cherished walks in nature. When asked how she felt about *that*, her response, again, was "sad."   This prompted Rick to somewhat playfully dub her knees "sad knees."   After only a few more rounds of tapping with the group, Jodi felt her tears shift inexplicably to laughter, prompting her to re-dub her knees "happy knees."

She was flabbergasted to learn that her new happy knees could walk up the stairs without any discomfort! At first she attributed this to the temporary relief one sometimes gets from FM. But as the workshop continued, she began to toy with the forbidden idea that her knees might heal completely. At one point, the whole group went for a nature walk and she found herself, without realizing it, leading the group. That was when she realized a life of pain was behind her.

Rick points out that a common problem with people who have a pain-intensive condition such as FM is that they become "human doings" (rather than human beings), in order to divert attention from the pain. Jodi fit that profile – she was a *very* productive person (except when it came to her own writing). It seemed that she would need to *slow down* and really learn to listen to her body if she wanted to sustain her progress. By developing a supportive relationship with her body, Rick felt she could use tapping as an ongoing tool for self-soothing and achieve continued mastery over the FM. He worked with her along those lines, and she responded beautifully.

Rick also was aware that Jodi had long allowed others to set the priorities for her life. As he put it, "she had a long list of people she was doing things for, but Jodi wasn't even on the list." He describes a major shift in her when she learned to put herself at the top of that list.

As for her relationship with writing, Jodi describes that transformation herself in her own new book! It is called *Tapping Into Clarity* (See Reference Section for details). In it she recounts the tapping session with Carol Look that triggered a shift in her writing life from blocked to bountiful. In a moment of insight, Jodi realized that she had been holding onto deep feelings of unworthiness around an issue with her daughter when the child was 13. Once she was able to recognize this and let it go, she gave herself "permission" to be successful. The words began flowing freely onto paper and have not stopped.

After

Jodi describes the four-day tapping workshop as a "life-changing event" for her. She experienced relief from her knee pain almost immediately – right after she tapped on it in the workshop. And the pain did not return. This experience seems to qualify as a bona fide One-Minute Wonder. But, of course, the big question was, "Will it last?'

In Jodi's case, the answer seems to be most emphatically "yes." She reports that she is currently pain-free and "up and down the stairs all day long." As testament to the transformation, she and her husband recently started building a two-story house, something she thought she would never be able to do again.

Equally as amazing, says Jodi, she regularly sleeps through the night now. Every morning she wakes up, shakes her head in disbelief, and says to herself, "Can you *believe* it?!" She adds, "If you had fibromyalgia, you'd know how incredible that is."

Jodi worked to release the sadness and the guilt of feeling as if she was not able to prevent her daughter's HIV. Jodi was able to forgive herself and to realize she did the best she knew how. This realization turned Jodi's life around. She was able to forgive and love herself again. This has transformed her family life and the way she reacts to her family. The Christmas after the workshop ended up being the most peaceful Christmas she has ever had with her family.

As for her writing career: as astounding as this may sound, she has not only completed one book, but three, within two months of leaving the workshop.

The key for Jodi – an important point to note – is that she continued tapping regularly after the workshop. She said she recognized that she had a golden opportunity and was not going to allow it to pass her by. She *knew* she had to make meridian tapping part of her life. She now taps every morning as part of her daily routine, tapping for abundance and other positive benefits. She also taps whenever a negative feeling comes up. "No sense storing it and having it come up later as an illness. Take care of it now. Tap all day long, tap whenever you can." Jodi has her whole family tapping now.

She has even become a meridian tapping practitioner herself and frequently uses the technique with others. Her husband, for example, recently had an eye condition no one could seem to properly diagnose. He'd been to four different doctors and still the inflammation persisted. As she and her husband were tapping together about it, he discovered that anger seemed to be at the root of the problem. Once he made that discovery and tapped on it, the next morning the eye problem was gone. It has not returned.

Jodi's plans for the near future are to become a bestselling author and to continue spreading the word about meridian tapping. With her attitude and commitment, who can doubt that she'll make it happen?

Jodi's Progress

Before:

- Pain in Knees.
- Pain in wrists.
- Could not go hiking.
- Could not ride a bike.
- Could not climb stairs.
- Diagnosed with insomnia.
- Took prescription Sonata.
- Took over the counter sleeping aids.
- Took steroid shots for knee pain.
- Took NSAIDs.
- Tried to write a book for 30 years with no success.

After:

- No pain in knees.
- No pain in wrists.
- Can go hiking.
- Bought a new bike and can go biking.
- No trouble walking up stairs – is building a house with two floors!
- No trouble sleeping.
- No longer needs sleeping aids.
- No longer needs NSAIDs.
- No longer needs steroid shots.
- Has no symptoms of fimbromyalgia.
- Wrote three books within 2 months after the event.

Chapter 21

Jon's Story

Before

Jonathan is a medically retired Vietnam veteran who now spends much of his time doing charity work. He applied for participation in the workshop in hopes that it would help him with a constellation of problems he'd been enduring for most of his adult life.

The most immediate and ever-present of these issues was his serious back pain. Jon had an accident back in 1974 which resulted in a severely herniated disc. He'd had four surgeries thus far to help correct the problem and had lived in more-or-less constant pain for over thirty years. There were other issues on the medical front as well. He had extreme tinnitus (ringing in the ears), high blood pressure, and sleep problems. On his application he reported that until recently he had not had a full night's sleep since he was a soldier in Vietnam in 1968. He also had diabetes, which he'd learned was a direct result of exposure to Agent Orange, and had recently suffered three mini-strokes that left him with numbness in parts of his face and hands.

Though his physical issues were daunting to say the least, perhaps even more devastating were the emotional and psychological scars from his years in Vietnam. Jon suffered PTSD following the Vietnam conflict and along with that disorder had come many years of nightmares, sleeplessness and relationship struggles. Jon has been married three times.

Though the tapping workshop group came to know Jon as a gentle man with an easy smile, this was not his usual demeanor at home. According to his wife Pearl, "Before the event I would describe Jon as grumpy. When the kids would come home they would find me and ask, 'Where's Dad?' That way, they knew to lower their voices or tiptoe around him." She further added, "He never laughed before the event; he was in too much pain." Jon himself acknowledged that before tapping he did not like being home for long periods of time and would frequently feel an anxious need to return to Vietnam.

Listening to Jon before and during the four-day workshop, it was clear that he suffered a great deal of guilt from the actions he had to carry out in the war. He described firing missiles and laughing as if it were a game – just one of the many mental tricks soldiers played to convince themselves they weren't killing real people. After four decades, Jon still hung his head in shame and sadness when he recalled certain details of the war. On an intellectual level, he knew he'd only been following orders, but on an emotional level, he felt great personal guilt. He also still bore a great deal of anger toward the elected officials whom he feels "duped" the country and young men such as himself into committing atrocious acts for dubious reasons.

Jon is a man who "puts his money where his mouth is." He has spent a great deal of time in Vietnam doing charity work, such as teaching. It is clear that Jonathan feels a deep debt to the people and the society he inadvertently harmed and disrupted during the war. He has great affection, respect and admiration for the Vietnamese people and has made helping them an important focus of his life's work.

Jon had never heard of meridian tapping until the day he filled out the workshop application. When asked why he wanted to participate, he replied, "I am eager to find a solution to my problems. I keep looking for something new and will try it." He added, "My area of focus is in helping people. I need to be in good physical health to continue what I am doing."

Jonathan was "very excited" about the possibility of participating in the program.

During

A striking aspect of Jon's experience in the four-day tapping retreat is that one of his most dramatic outcomes revolved around a phobia not even mentioned in his application materials. Jon had an intense and abiding fear of rats.

Unlike many phobias, which tend to have an irrational foundation, Jon's fear of rats was sickeningly well-grounded in reality. In Vietnam, says Jon:

> We slept in underground bunkers to protect us from surprise mortar attacks at night. I was sleeping one night when I felt something heavy on my leg. I shone the flashlight on it and saw a huge rat the size of a cat. I kicked it off of my leg and spent the rest of the night outside. The next day we tore the bunker down and found the rat and its nest.
>
> That night I went to another bunker and as I'm getting ready to sleep I see *another* rat. I grabbed an iron rod and tried to kill it. It crawled into a hole in the sandbags and I was ramming it with the rod trying to kill it. I looked into the hole and it jumped out at me. I ducked and it landed on my bed. I was trying to hit it with the rod, but it kept trying to get me. I was finally able to kill it.

From that point on, Jon says, he was so afraid of rats, he would sneak his cot out of the bunker every night and sleep outside. He was less afraid of mortar-fire than he was of the rats.

Since his Vietnam days, Jon had sustained an aversion to rats that was so strong he could not speak about them without intense anxiety – it was a full-blown phobia. In the workshop, just asking Jon to think about rats brought him to a ten on the intensity scale.

Steve, the staff person who worked most closely with Jonathan, describes going through a fairly standard, and very successful, phobia "treatment" with Jon for his rat fears. Typically, this involves doing multiple rounds of tapping during which the intensity is gradually lessened, along with tapping on as many

Aspects of the fear as the person can uncover. With Jon's rat fears, there were many *Aspects*. In addition to his frightening close-encounters was his aversion to seeing the creatures feeding on the bodies of dead soldiers, the fear of infection and disease, the appearance and disturbing habits of the creatures, etc.

Astonishingly, by the end of the four-day workshop Jon was able to literally hold a live rat on his lap with no problem at all (one was brought into the workshop). He was also able to view a film of the very bunker in Vietnam where the rats had been, without any emotional reaction to seeing it — for the very first time.

Conquering his fear of rats had important implications for Jon. Fears and phobias can have a debilitating effect on many people and especially on men who view themselves as "warriors." In Jon's case, he had certainly transformed himself into a *peaceful* warrior through his charity work in Vietnam. But still, the persistent fear of rats was a constant, weakening drain on his self-perception. Now he could return to the villages of that country with more confidence, no longer terrified by these animals.

The disappearance of Jon's back pain was no less dramatic. As Steve worked with him around this issue, he learned that, as a child, Jon had been beaten repeatedly by his father on the back with a heavy leather strap. Jon talks about this in the film. As Jon tapped about this, a picture emerged of a boy who had been frequently whipped and beaten by his father but who had received little or no outward love from him. Jon had borne this burden "on his back" for years and carried the pain, literally, into adulthood. During the workshop Jon tapped on various emotions and events related to his father and, in doing so, could practically *feel* the back pain dissipating. Before the workshop was over, he was sitting cross-legged on the floor, a position he'd been unable to get into for many, many years, and he was reporting that he was pain free.

Jon also made great strides with his guilt. It seems that during his many post-war visits to Vietnam, Jon was involved in bringing families back to the U.S. Each time he was unable to succeed with a particular family, he took it *very* hard and very personally. Jon came to realize that no matter how much he did, it was never enough for him. He was a bottomless pit in this regard. So deep was his guilt from the war that he wanted to save the whole country, in a sense (but of course could not). At the workshop he was able to recognize this pattern and to tap into greater insight about it.

His most important insight of all, perhaps, was this: he realized that he had been unable to allow *himself* a happy family life because he felt he had ruined so many families in Vietnam. Simply by having this realization, he says, he has been able to transform that part of his life.

After

The follow-up report on Jonathan is, by necessity, brief. Why? Well, because it was difficult to reach him after the workshop. You see, he went back to Vietnam to teach.

Teach what? Meridian tapping. Jon has taught his Vietnamese friends how to use the technique for many different life challenges. It has been extremely well-received there. One of the main uses has been with teenagers dealing with anxiety over school exams.

But probably the most significant aspect of his last trip to Vietnam was that he chose to cut it short in order to come home and be with his own family. This was something he'd never done before.

His relationship with his wife and children has dramatically improved since the workshop. He finds himself smiling and laughing around the house and enjoying the time he spends there, rather than getting anxious to leave. His daughter puts it this way, "I feel like Dad is a new person. I love this new person."

In the months since the four-day retreat, Jon has been virtually free of back pain. Remember that this pain had been a constant and debilitating companion in his life. As for the rats – Jon was in a restaurant during his last trip to Vietnam when one of these rodents scurried across the floor. Jon says that he observed the event unemotionally. The power of tapping to help free him of daily back pain, along with the enormous emotional benefits he has derived from the practice, have convinced Jon that meridian tapping is a wonderful, healing gift to bring back to the land and people he has come to love so much.

But he is also sharing the gift here at home. Jon plans to spend the summer of 2008 teaching meridian tapping at veterans' shelters and to people in the VA.

What more needs to be said? Congratulations and thanks to you, Jonathan.

Jon's Progress

Before:

- Severe back pain for 15 years.
- Extreme fear of rats.
- Didn't like spending time at home.
- Felt he could never have a happy family because he had ruined other families through participation in the Viet Nam war.
- Was spending months at a time in Vietnam volunteering out of guilt.
- Rarely laughed. His wife said, "He never laughed before, he was in too much pain."

After:

- Back pain is gone. "I sometimes feels a little ache in my back and I begin to tap and it goes away. The severe pain I had before is gone".
- No longer has fear of rats. Held a rat.
- Brought meridian tapping to Vietnam to help others.
- Went to Vietnam and cut the trip short to go home and spend time with his family.
- Enjoys being at home with his family.
- He no longer volunteers in Vietnam out of guilt. "I go because I love the people."
- "He smiles and laughs!" says his wife Pearl.

Chapter 22

Patricia's Story

Before

Patricia had always been, in her own words, a "healthy, active" person. She loved the outdoors and enjoyed physical activities like yoga, hiking and cycling. So it was not surprising that, on a first date with a man she'd just met, she found herself skimming across the waves in a boat, soaking in the fresh air and sunshine.

What was *totally unexpected* was what happened next. "One minute I'm on a boat, the next minute I'm lying in an emergency room... and they're telling me I can't walk." Patricia simply could not make sense of the news the ER team was trying to communicate to her – that her back had been broken and she needed emergency surgery in order to save her legs, bowel and bladder.

Evidently she'd been in a freak boating accident. But how and when had it happened? No time had passed for her since she was standing on a boat deck, riding the swells and feeling the cool spray on her face.

Later she would recall a single flash of memory – lying on the floor of the boat at a horrible angle, knocked out of her own shoes, and feeling hot waves of anger toward the man who'd been at the helm, for speeding the boat so fast. But now she was lying on a bed in the ER, no idea how she'd gotten there, and in "pain that took my breath away." She describes the suddenness of the experience as "scary... weird... almost unbelievable."

It turned out Patricia had shattered her L1, one of the large lumbar vertebrae of the lower back.

Her surgery was "successful," but resulted in a repair job that included four titanium rods and eight sets of screws and bolts around the fracture site, incorporating the three vertebrae above and below the broken one. She was warned by her treatment team that she would always suffer some degree of pain and discomfort and that she would live a compromised life as a result of the injury and surgery.

The accident was as much a blow to Patricia's self-image as her body. Not only had she always been physically active, but, as a product of a military upbringing, she had always seen herself as capable, upbeat and confident, with a "you can do anything" attitude. She now had to ask her employer for time off and rely on family members for help and care. She did not want to be thought of as the "girl with the back pain." Never having been one to feel defeated or to use pain as an excuse, she now found herself dealing with pain so intense she sometimes thought, "I don't know if I can continue living if this is what it'll be like."

On her application form for the workshop, and prior to trying meridian tapping, Patricia describes her life after the accident: "It still feels like I'm living a bad dream that I'll wake up out of.... Everything has been modified... and I'm still adapting, adjusting, trying to find the right balance." She adds, "I hate that I always have to ask 'how will this activity/event/decision affect my back?' I'm much slower than I used to be and that's frustrating. I'm afraid that people may perceive my situation as being handicapped. The accident has totally redefined my life and I resent that but try to focus on the positive."

After the accident, Patricia was determined *not* to be defined by her injury and not to allow the somber predictions of medical professionals to limit her recovery. She refused to dwell on the pain and constantly searched for new treatments, new points of view, and new types of therapy that might offer promise. One day she came across an article that showed a link between cancer and trauma. It scared her.

That was all she needed, she thought, cancer on top of everything else! Scrambling to dig up more information, she recalled having seen a notice about a new kind of trauma treatment on Dr. Joseph Mercola's holistic health website. She followed the link to the tapping workshop site, read about the four-day workshop program, and almost immediately knew, "I need to do this."

Although there were over a hundred applicants to the program, Patricia was selected to participate. She arrived on Day One, a little late and in back pain that was telling her she should had flown instead of driving, but filled with optimism. Maybe this new technique called meridian tapping would help her deal with "this hardware in my back" that had radically altered her life.

Patricia was ready to make it work or at least give it an open-minded effort. "You never know until you try. What have I got to lose?" was the way she felt.

During

A striking aspect of Patricia's participation in the workshop was that she seemed to feel her issues were "minor" compared with those of others. It was a bit surprising to some of the participants that she did not view her severe physical trauma as being on a par with the issues they were grappling with. Taking note of this, the meridian tapping team made sure to give a great deal of respect and importance to Patricia's body issues as they worked with her around them.

As she tapped, it became clear that she had strong feelings that she "shouldn't have been there" on the boat when the accident occurred. She did not like motor boats and at that point did not yet know or trust the man she was with. She felt she had gone against her gut instincts and was somehow paying the price for that.

Much of her tapping work involved tapping through the accident and its aftermath with thoroughness and diligence, paying particular attention to the moments when she received the traumatic news about her back and the dire prognostications. She tapped about the limiting beliefs that were held by others and herself about her injury. Tapping through the many *Aspects* of the accident and the healing process brought noticeable relief to Patricia.

One key strategy the team used was to have Patricia tap on accepting the man-made materials that had been implanted in her back as "the new normal." As Rick points out, the human brain has not evolved quickly enough to regard foreign objects implanted in the body as non-threatening. Without some active retraining, it tends to regard such materials in the same way it would an arrow or a blade. The meridian tapping facilitators worked to help Patricia "re-tune" her mind/body so she could think of her artificial "hardware" as normal and non-threatening.

As a result, Patricia's pain dramatically decreased and her mind was able to easily shift its focus away from the foreign materials in her back.

After

Patricia's progress since the workshop has been nothing short of remarkable. Before trying meridian tapping she had been constantly aware of her back. She describes the physical feeling as having been one of "weightiness," as if she were carrying a heavy battery pack or a brick on her lower back. In winter, it got worse and "felt like someone had swung a bat at it."

But more than the pain itself had been the constant *awareness* of the injury and the planning and adapting around it.

Now, six months after the workshop, Patricia actually has trouble remembering that she has an injury. For instance, when Jackie met her for the reunion in April, she kept offering to carry Patricia's bags. Patricia didn't understand why and finally had to remind herself about her own injury. "I don't think about my back most of the time... It's almost like it never happened," she says. When she does think about it, "It feels more matter-of-fact." She no longer finds herself planning her life around her pain and mobility issues. Even the weighty feeling in the lower back is absent. Pain no longer defines her daily life. Her sense of identity has shifted away from the injury.

Perhaps even more gratifying have been the emotional benefits Patricia reports from having done tapping regularly, "I feel calmer and happier about things." Thinking back on the injury, the surgery, and the painful recovery she says, "I feel at peace with the whole process."

She describes a new sense of acceptance, evenness and equanimity that was not present before discovering meridian tapping. For example, she formerly felt extremely uncomfortable asking people for help, even approaching her employer for time off after the accident. Now she wonders, "Why? What was the big deal? I had broken my *back*!"

Probably the most dramatic shift has been around her feelings of anger. After the accident and prior to the tapping workshop, Patricia felt "rage" toward the man who'd been driving the boat, a man she'd only just met. In the ensuing three years since she'd last seen him, her rage continued to fester. "Why did he have to go so fast?" she would ruminate, over and over. It got to the point where she dreaded the thought of ever seeing the man again, should their case go to court. The idea filled her with anxiety.

Then one day, a few months after the tapping workshop, she was walking down the street in Washington D.C., when she spotted a group of businessmen walking together. One of them caught her eye and she realized it was him – the man who had caused her accident. Patricia was wearing sunglasses and walked past the group without his even noticing her. And how did she feel about the near encounter? "After all that tapping, I felt neutral," she reports. There was no anger, no anxiety. It was "no big deal."

When it comes to the rage, Patricia says, "Now, to me, there's no value in being angry. It doesn't matter anymore." And she says it with a peaceful calm in her voice that's hard to contradict. This feeling has been neutralized, it no longer controls her.

Patricia has made tapping a regular part of her life ever since she learned the method in October. This is an important point. She will often tap when faced with an emotional or physical challenge and finds that each time this brings her to a new level in her personal development. Had she stopped the use of tapping right after the workshop, it is doubtful if she would have benefited in nearly as profound a fashion as she has.

If there is a "moral" to her story, it is that with meridian tapping, persistence and dedication can pay off beautifully.

Patricia's Progress

Before:

- Extreme back pain.
- Took morphine, Percocet, Norco, and Valium.
- Trouble sleeping.
- Took Ambien for sleep.
- Inability to travel for work without taking advance measures.
- Inability to hike without brace.
- Could not do Vinyasa yoga.
- Anger towards man who drove boat.
- Anxiety over hospital and medical tests.
- Trouble asking others for help.

After:

- No longer has any back pain.
- No longer takes any prescription medicine.
- No longer has trouble sleeping.
- No longer needs sleep medicine.
- Can travel without thinking about back.
- Can hike comfortably without brace.
- Did yoga challenges by taking yoga every day for 22 days.
- No longer has anger over accident and driver.
- Relieved anxiety over medical tests.
- Ask others for help without feeling embarrassed.

Chapter 23

Rene's Story

Before

Rene came to the workshop through a slightly different route than the other participants. It seems that Nick and Jessica, the organizers/producers, were motivated to ensure that the participant pool reflected a robust ethnic, racial, age and gender diversity. As they approached filming date, they became concerned that it was not *quite* as diverse as they had hoped.

Jessica took matters into her own hands and traveled to Harlem, New York, where she spent a day handing out flyers and talking about the movie in a heavily minority-populated neighborhood. She had many interesting encounters, but no real takers. As she walked down a street she saw a phone booth with a torn-up paper on it. Although she was well aware that you're not allowed to cover phone booths with flyers, she put two workshop fliers on two phone booths next to each other. Those were the only two fliers she put up in Harlem; she just "felt" like she should.

Those two phone booths were right across from Rene's brother's restaurant. As Rene was leaving that day the flyer caught his eye and he too just "felt" like he should apply. To this day they both feel they were "guided" on that Sunday afternoon.

When the team heard Rene's story, they moved quickly to accept him into the program, even though he had not gone through the same acceptance process as the other applicants. The next day Jessica and Nick Polizzi drove to his house to interview him. This is now the footage you see at the beginning of the movie.

About two and half months earlier, Rene had been in a car accident. Traveling in the car with him were his wife and soulmate, Raquel, plus a couple of her children from a previous marriage. No drugs or alcohol were involved. Rene was observing all safety rules and had, in fact, only moments earlier, instructed one of the children to put his safety belt on. Their car collided with a truck that was merging onto the highway and was demolished. Rene and the children were injured, but Raquel was killed instantly.

Rene was devastated. His life since the accident had been, essentially, one long, uninterrupted shock reaction. He constantly replayed "tapes in his head" from the accident over and over, hundreds of times a day. He felt enormous guilt at somehow, magically, not having been able to avert the accident. Opposed to suicide for religious reasons, he often found himself just lying on the floor for hours, wishing it all would end.

Raquel was the mother of six children from a previous marriage, the youngest two of which Rene was helping her raise. After the accident the two children returned to Puerto Rico to be with their biological father. The house that had been filled with a loving wife and two young, energetic children was now empty and quiet. Rene's life had been turned inside out and upside down. He was numb, spinning his tires, going nowhere. He could not move on.

When the film crew visited his home, they found a veritable "shrine" that Rene had constructed for Raquel. Photos and memorabilia were carefully placed in groupings all around the apartment, ensuring that Rene literally could not open his eyes without being reminded of his late, beloved "Kelly."

He came to the workshop out of desperation but with no real hope that it would make much of a difference. In his mind his life was over and he would never be happy again. Yet something inside of him told him to give it a try.

During

If you saw the film, *The Tapping Solution*, you undoubtedly recall one of its most jarring and poignant scenes. Rene was describing the "Oh my God!" moment his mind kept replaying as he recalled the instant before the crash. When asked to voice the words with their true emotional power, Rene's intensity leaped instantly from a 1 to a 10 and he shouted "OH MY GOD!" in visceral shock and horror. It was *this* moment, with *this* intensity, that kept intruding on Rene's consciousness hour after hour, day after day.

It was easy for the meridian tapping facilitators to see why he was having trouble "moving on."

The team also learned about another aspect of the accident that lent it even more tragedy. Rene and his wife Raquel, as mentioned above, were raising children from her previous marriage but had no children of their own. Only moments before the accident, however, Raquel had suddenly informed him that she thought she might be pregnant with *their* first child. One can only imagine how this news impacted him at the time he was driving and had further added to the grief and guilt he was experiencing.

The meridian tapping team helped Rene focus on specific memory *Aspects* of the accident and its aftermath in order to try to reduce the intensity and frequency of the intrusive thoughts. They also worked with him around the guilt he felt. Rene shared with the team that he and his wife had frequently argued in their marriage, both being high intensity, passionate people. This was another reason he felt so guilty. Her forgiveness for their various arguments had never been given to him. He flip-flopped between anger and guilt during much of the workshop.

At one point, Rene described a dent Raquel had put in his car with her fist during one of their arguments. Helena asked him to take her out to his car (not the same car that had been in the accident). She tapped with him as they looked at and touched the actual dent. Rene could not remember the content of the argument they'd been having, but the dent stood as a constant reminder of their arguing. Helena encouraged him to use the dent, instead, as a reminder to forgive himself. Rene cried at this, but as they continued tapping, his tears turned to a smile. He realized, he said, that Raquel was somehow present "in the dent," that she wasn't really gone. There seemed to be a genuine shift in his bearing and facial expression from that moment on.

In some of the more memorable moments of the workshop, fellow participants recall Rene dancing and playing the drums with a new playfulness and lightness in his eyes. He had not finished his grieving process by any means, but something had shifted for him.

After

Since the workshop, Rene has regained the ability to sleep at night. He no longer needs to leave the TV on to fill the emptiness. He has started a new business venture and is excited about it. He has also begun a workout plan and has lost 15 pounds. The ability to set goals and follow through on them shows a healthy integration and cohesion in Rene that was not present when he came to the workshop.

Perhaps the most meaningful change is that the intensity and intrusiveness of the crash memories have subsided. "With tapping I was able to quiet the noise in my head," says Rene. "Now I feel so much closer to Raquel." When asked to elaborate on this, Rene explains that he and his wife had shared a deep spiritual connection when she was alive. After the accident, though, the noise of his intrusive thoughts and memories was so loud, it drowned out her spiritual presence. Since doing tapping, Rene says he has been able to dramatically "turn down the volume" on the inner noise and thereby reconnect with her on a spiritual level. Spirit speaks in stillness and quiet.

Rene still grieves and misses Raquel everyday. He continues to tap consistently with Jessica by phone. He realized that he believed he never wanted to stop feeling pain because his pain meant that he was remembering Raquel. With some tapping on this belief he came to his own conclusion, "The best way to honor her is to enjoy life and smile, because that is what she always did." Although Rene is still grieving, everyday he makes major strides in his life. "If the negative feelings come up I tap and then I feel in control again," say Rene. Rene looks forward to growing his business and buying a house in Puerto Rico. Rene's friends and family are happy to see his big smile and hear his joyous laugh again.

Rene's Progress

Before:

- Constantly replayed the memory of the accident.
- Felt guilt over the accident.
- Felt guilt about fighting with Raquel in the past.
- Could not sleep without the television.
- Could not be motivated to do work.
- Could not be motivated to work out.
- Could not make any plans for the future.

After:

- No longer consistently plays the accident.
- Can think about the accident without feeling intense emotions.
- No longer feels guilt over the accident.
- No longer feels guilt about fighting with Raquel.
- Went back to work.
- Started a second business venture.
- Began to work out again.
- Lost 15 lbs.
- Can make plans for the future – is planning to grow business and buy a house is Puerto Rico.
- Is smiling and laughing again!

Chapter 24

Sam's Story

Before

Sam is an intelligent and motivated young man who, for years, had been dealing with a baffling and debilitating complex of physical disorders that had been affecting his life profoundly.

At the top of the list were his frequent and intense headaches. "My head feels as if there was a 500-pound anvil pushing it down. It has lots of pressure and feels like it will explode." He described extreme sensitivity and soreness throughout his sinus system. "My eyes constantly sting and feel as if they are going to pop out."

Sam further reported, "I am always feeling tired, as if I am in need of a nap. Every morning I feel like my body weighs a thousand pounds and I am not very coherent. It is very tough to wake up and start the day regardless of how much sleep I get. I live off my adrenaline every day."

On his application form Sam supplied a long list of other physical symptoms that included sore muscles, swollen extremities, tightness and burning in the lungs, a mysterious dark blue/grey plaque around his inner thigh, bladder problems, stomach pains, throat discomfort and constriction, bowel issues, and a strange inability to gain weight, despite the fact that he was always hungry and could "eat a horse."

One of the main effects his symptoms were having on his life was that, "My brain is all foggy and it is very difficult to read, think, ponder, or study for normal amounts of time." Concentration and focus were noticeably lacking. His mental life was suffering tremendously.

Sam describes his problems as starting in high school. "I lived a very busy life as a senior and had irregular sleep patterns. I did not get lots of sleep so I thought that that was the main reason that I was always tired. I also fell asleep very easily and began to feel foggy-headed."

A couple of years later, following a service mission to El Salvador for his church, Sam was diagnosed with Viral-Spinal Meningitis and CMV and EBV viruses. However, there had also been, and continued to be, many symptoms that these diagnoses could not account for. "Doctors have passed me along to other doctors and finally have suggested that they cannot help me and that I should learn to deal with it, and so I have."

Reading Sam's history of physical disorders, along with his experiences of these, one can't help feeling that his somatic issues have more complex roots than have yet been uncovered. In the months leading up to the tapping workshop, Sam had incurred large medical bills, due to lack of health insurance, and had continued to receive complicated and baffling diagnoses. In one incident, for example, he said, "I pretty much slept for four days until my throat was so tight I could not eat or drink for three days. I became dehydrated and finally decided to go to the ER. I ended up getting an endoscopy to find out that I had three viral infections in my esophagus and a sepsis in my bloodstream."

Sam listed a partial sampling of about fifteen specialists he had seen, including not only Western medical doctors but acupuncturists, Chinese herbalists, cranial masseurs, chiropractors and "several energy doctors." He described his current condition: "I still suffer from the heavy headaches, burning pain, sore/stiff muscles, tight/inflamed lungs, stomach/bowels pain, constipation, weak immune system, extreme fatigue, etc. I have to make the decision every day to wake up and charge forward. It's either stay in bed and cry or wake up and live off my adrenaline all day."

It's important to note, though, that Sam does not see himself as a victim. Prior to the workshop he reported, "I believe that my overall happiness is in my control. I choose how I react and what I learn from experiences." Sam presents himself as a positive, high-energy person who sings, plays soccer and has started his own non-profit self-development venture called "Overcome to Become." "The primary focus in my life," he writes, "has been increasing the wellbeing and happiness of others. I love to help others be happy. I have always been the guy who gets people together for good times." Sam sought out the tapping workshop in the hope that he could regain his mental concentration and find some way to ease the pain and fatigue from the headaches and numerous other symptoms. Anticipating the workshop he said, "Wow! My life would be a whole new world if I did not have this health problem. I would be so much more effective. It would help me reach my many goals and aspirations and I could enjoy life at a whole new level. I would love that!"

During

In many ways, Sam was perhaps the most consistently challenging of the workshop participants. Though he did experience periods of relief from the pain, as well as some genuine "a-ha!" moments of insight and clarity, he also experienced moments of increased pain intensity. There were more ups and downs with Sam than is typical of someone learning tapping in a workshop environment,

This is not surprising, given the very serious physical imbalances that Sam was dealing with. Rick believes that ups and downs are often signs of an imbalanced body *trying to come into balance*. But, says Rick, Sam had not yet gained the "energetic and emotional foundation with which to stand at a different level and hold that consistently."

There seems to be agreement among the program staff that Sam did have some meaningful glimpses and "openings" into what a more balanced life would feel like, but that he would need a longer period of sustained, structured work in order to make lasting changes. At this time in his life, Sam is a young man with a busy social life, a lot of friends and a "big persona." It may be that his life does not currently lend itself to the slow, sustained inner work of finding bodily and emotional balance. Right now, Sam's strategy – not necessarily a bad one – has been to focus on other things and to keep himself busy rather than to consciously face the intensity of his physical pain with both eyes open and a willingness to encounter it, whatever the cost.

The meridian tapping facilitators believe Sam has emotional issues he was not completely ready to deal with openly. Steve, who worked most closely with him, feels that at his deepest core, shame is a great burden for Sam.

Just the fact that his physical pain could *have* an emotional component seemed like a revelation to Sam, so it is not surprising that he was not fully ready to work on it at that level. As Rick points out, though, when someone comes to a healing milieu to work on physical pain, but is not correspondingly ready and able to work on the *emotional* pain, success will always be limited.

Rick's sense about Sam is that the progress he *was* able to make, in areas such as improved focus, came about as a result of partial "entrainment" of the "head and heart." Head/heart entrainment creates "in the zone"-type experiences and lowers stress and pain. Rick believes that further ongoing head/heart work would bring Sam great benefits and longer-lasting results.

After

Sam's most obvious benefit from the workshop was his increased ability to concentrate.

"My mom was even impressed with how I could study and stay focused when I got back from the retreat," he reports.

At this point, the workshop staff feels that Sam would benefit from a longer-term commitment to inner work. Like all the participants Sam had the opportunity to work with Jessica Ortner by telephone approximately once a week, but he kept missing his appointments. Finally it was decided that he would no longer get the coaching because of his lack of commitment. Sam agreed that he was too busy. Recently, however, Jessica did speak to him. She reports, "Although Sam has horrible pain he has learned to function efficiently with it. Because of this he doesn't look at healing the pain as his number one priority." Sam echoes this, saying, "I have trained myself to run away from how I physically feel. I think that's why I haven't gone back to tapping – because it means I have to take time and feel the feelings. I'm right back to my crazy busy life but I realize that I need to go back to tapping. I will when the time comes. I think I'm just not ready right now." Reportedly, he does still use tapping occasionally for improving his concentration and finds it helpful in that regard. That alone is progress. His pain has not noticeably decreased, however. But, again, he is not tapping for that benefit, nor is he tapping consistently.

In all, our picture of Sam is a mixed one – partial "success" for the retreat and for tapping, and partial "failure." This is not a surprising outcome for participants new to meridian tapping, though in this regard Sam is definitely in the minority among the ten workshop participants. The majority clearly benefited, often in a marked and surprising manner. What Sam's case indicates is that tapping is not "magic"; it cannot work when there is not full readiness for it to do its job. In this respect, tapping is no different from any other healing modality, whether traditional or alternative. The person must be in a certain "place" in his or her own life to benefit from it, and in the final analysis the choice belongs to the person.

Sam's Progress

Before:

- Extreme difficulty focusing and studying – "foggy brain".
- Severe headaches.
- Sore/Stiff muscles.
- Extreme fatigue.
- "I feel like my body weighs a thousand pounds".
- Inflamed lungs.
- Throat constriction.
- Stomach/bowel pains.

After

- No longer has difficulty focusing and studying.
- Severe headaches.
- Sore/Stiff muscles.
- Extreme fatigue.
- Physical symptoms, in general, not improved.

Thea's Story

Before

One of the most difficult conditions mental health counselors are called upon to treat is a serious addiction. It takes high professional skill, specialized training, persistence, and a strong support system to protect the addicted person from succumbing to the overwhelming lure of what, for them, seems to be a "solution." After all, they have found something that "works" for them, something that seems to solve a host of unbearable problems. It is not easy for an emotionally threatened person to give up what seems to be their only safety net.

Thea, one of the participants in the four-day workshop, falls into this category. She had been suffering from powerful multiple addictions. She is a 22-year-old mom who described herself when she applied for the workshop, in the following way, "I have a severely addictive personality — whether it's prescription drugs, food or Diet Coke, I don't know the meaning of the word moderation… Furthermore, I have extremely low self-esteem, a VERY hard time keeping my word to myself and others, a chronically hard time keeping my house clean, and I battle depression."

Keeping her word was therefore extremely hard for Thea as it is for so many addictive personalities – and it can be their downfall. Thea had been diagnosed (incorrectly, she says) with ADD in her early-to-mid-teens and placed on the medication Adderall, which she stayed on until she was about 20, "at which point I started abusing prescription pain killers (Percocet) and alcohol, which I did up until 1½ months ago." At that time, Thea entered detox and began a prescription Methadone program.

So Thea had only very recently left the worst of her addictive substances behind her when she came to the four-day retreat. She was just *beginning* the difficult road of recovery. This is important to note because social scientists have recently discovered that the traditional notion that addicts should be rushed into ACTION with regard to "kicking" their addiction before they may be inwardly ready to do so, is actually in error. It seems there is a series of inner steps that *must* be taken first, a "readiness" that must occur, before there is a serious chance for such a program to be successful. These steps are now being incorporated into many anti-addiction programs.

The six-step process is described in the book, *Changing for Good*, by James Prochaska, John Norcross and Carlo DiClemente. According to these authors, one's ability to change is directly related to these stages of inner development: precontemplation, contemplation, preparation, action, maintenance and termination. To fail to go through *any one* of these stages can be a prescription for failure – steps cannot be skipped.

In a fascinating CD program, meridian tapping experts Carol Look and David Rourke discuss the six steps in terms of their implications for using tapping to conquer addiction. Meridian tapping, they point out, must be applied strategically to *each one of the stages* in turn. In their audio program, Look and Rourke lead the listener through a number of targeted tapping strategies that they can use for this purpose, but always, *always* emphasize the importance of never rushing a person before they are fully ready for the next stage. It only backfires.

David Rourke, in fact, reports some terrifying statistics regarding programs that do not abide by this "readiness" principle. He cites studies that show that within *three hours* of discharge from a 28-day rehabilitation program, 90% of the participants had *already* relapsed – already partaken of their addictive substance. This is devastating evidence of the folly of moving too rapidly when dealing with addictions.

Thea "failed" to benefit from the four-day retreat after returning home, as you will see, although she showed some surprising benefits from using meridian tapping during the program itself. Clearly she was not yet ready for the huge challenge that giving up her addictions, and even the debilitating symptoms that accompanied them, entailed. Her experience is important because it so clearly demonstrates the limitations of any treatment, tapping included, if certain essential steps are not followed when dealing with addiction.

Thea did seem to be past the stage known as "precontemplation" where the addict denies any problems and is still blaming everyone else for criticizing their behavior. She was insightful on her admissions form when she described how her addiction issue had touched her life. "It has affected everything horribly. While I was abusing Adderall/Percocet/alcohol, I became very self-centered (which I'm still working on), lied, cheated, manipulated and stole, resulting in damaging most of my family and friend relationships. I was sexually abused when I was in my early teens, but with my past of lying so much, my family doesn't even believe that. As a result, I feel alone, constantly fearful and depressed. I want to break out of the cycle so badly, but on my own, it is very difficult."

We can see that a substantial part of Thea genuinely wanted to change. She described herself as "EXTREMELY EAGER" to work on her condition, "I want it more than anything else in the world." she said and stated that her baby son was her main focus in life and that her greatest fear was losing him, along with the possibility of being molested again.

But the fact is that another part of her was not yet ready for the very hard work of change, the discouragement an addicted person inevitably encounters along the way, and the great persistence required.

Thea had not heard of meridian tapping before she came to the retreat. In fact, it was her husband who did the research and recommended she try the workshop. This may have turned out to be a crucial factor in her response to the program and to tapping in general. Going for help because someone else wants it is not usually productive (see more on this in Dennis's story). However, Thea claimed to feel eager to participate in the workshop and was excited when she was invited to attend.

During

Helena was the meridian tapping practitioner who worked most closely with Thea. Helena freely admits that she is not an expert on working with addictions. She reports that, right from the start, however, she had an intuitive sense that Thea did not genuinely want help with her addictions. Thea *did* seem genuinely sick and tired of her life the way it was. She truly seemed to want to be a good mother to her baby boy and seemed to genuinely recognize the part she had played in alienating her family members. She was not blaming the world for her problems. Those were hopeful signs.

However, her ever-present can of Coke and several-times-daily purchases of candy bars and ice cream from the corner store were reminders that perhaps she was just in a place of trading one addiction for another.

Helena describes Thea as reluctant to share and "more guarded than anyone else." Her sense was that Thea was "not really living her own life." Like several of the other women in the workshop, Thea had trouble thinking of goals she wanted for herself. All of her goals revolved around being better for her son. She did not seem to claim any authentic ground for herself.

Thea did gain at least one concrete benefit from the tapping retreat. Like Jodi, she had suffered for some time from chronic, intense pain in the knees. She told of needing her husband to carry the baby downstairs in the morning, while she hobbled down, grasping the handrail. Because Jodi had already successfully conquered her own knee pain, she was asked to play the role of workshop leader and take Thea through some rounds of tapping. Not long after this session, Thea was bounding up the stairs, apparently pain-free.

Thea was also able to experience, in the words of Rick, a "culture of caring" she was not used to. Nothing in her previous experiences, including her addiction treatments, had seemingly prepared her for being fully accepted and cared about for who she was *right now*, with no subtle messages that she was undeserving of such good will.

Thea parted Clear Point in good spirits, apparently glad to have participated and happy to have made some personal connections.

After

Thea pulled back from the program staff upon her return home (participants were asked to maintain follow-up contacts). Although at first she answered the phone calls of team members, she soon ceased to do so and could not be contacted by them. It appears that she had not been successful in her addiction recovery. Given what we know about addictive behavior and the need for readiness to change, this seems the likeliest outcome. But we don't know for sure.

Why did Thea "fail," then?

Rick points out that the One-Minute-Wonders that often occur at meridian tapping events can create unrealistic expectations that everyone who tries this technique is supposed to be a quick-cure "star." Participants in any workshop can also get a "workshop high," which leads to false beliefs that everything can be fixed over the course of a long weekend. In fact, only a minority of problems clear up extremely rapidly, even with tapping. Serious issues, such as sexual abuse and addictions, take more time and attention. Thea would have benefited, says Rick, from much private one-on-one work and a long-term approach.

It should be noted that some of the team members had felt, right from the start, that Thea was not a good candidate for the workshop. The fact that she was on methadone alone signified to some that she was not yet at the point in her psycho-physiological recovery process where she could really make use of a self-help technique such as meridian tapping that demands self-discipline. Still, her participation, even if was not a textbook "success," was valuable in that it helps to illustrate the limits of any kind of treatment method, tapping included, when a person is not fully ready.

Thea's current avoidance of the program staff may not be an "escape." She may merely be regrouping internally, preparing for a next step. And who knows – perhaps the seeds of something powerful were indeed planted in Thea's life that weekend, seeds that will blossom and bear fruit when *Thea* is ready.

Thea's Progress

Before:

- Wanted help with "extreme addictive behavior".
- Had frequent nightmares.
- Was often dishonest.
- Had severe arthritis in her knees; was unable to pick up her son out of the crib in the morning and had trouble going up stairs.
- Extreme fatigue.

After:

- Still likely has severe addictive behavior.
- Nightmares are gone.
- Knee pain, which was "95% gone" after the workshop (and while Thea continued to tap) has now returned full-force.
- Low energy has returned.
- Dishonesty has resumed.

Thea has not been in contact with the production team for many months. However, her husband was able to provide some of the above information. He adds, "Tapping was really a miracle to her, it's so sad that she stopped."

PART 5

What to Expect

A doctor is often with the patient one or two hours a year. The patient is with the patient the other 8758 hours.

Recognizing the enormous healing powers of the body — and finding ways to engage them — presupposes an entirely different model from the classic image of the patient being fixed by a doctor or hospital.*

Dawson Church, Ph.D.
Researcher, Author, Expert in Energy Medicine

Tapping is likely to become a first line of defense for those seeking conventional medical treatment, in some instances it may avert the necessity for this treatment entirely.

*Quote from the book The Genie in Your Genes, by Dr. Dawson Church, one of the experts in the movie, *The Tapping Solution*.

Chapter 26

The Future of
Meridian Tapping

We stand at a turning point in human history. For the past three hundred years we have watched from the sidelines as human beings have been systematically dethroned from their position as the inspirational center of the cosmos to nothing more than a random collection of atoms animated by cold and impersonal natural laws. Isaac Newton's falling apple, while useful in many of its simpler applications, has dominated our thinking. Most of us were raised to believe that the human body is a machine, the heart is a pump and the reach of the human mind goes no further than the skull. What is real is what can be seen, heard and touched. Anything else is suspect.

The pendulum is swinging back. The discoveries we are making in physics, psychology, and medicine are showing us a world far more marvelous, complex and mysterious than any colliding-ball model could possibly explain. We now *know* that we live in a world of particles *and* waves. And the waves are the really interesting part. With each passing day, human beings are emerging more clearly as incredibly complex systems of energy fields, inextricably interwoven with one another and the world around us. Much of the majesty and mystery of human life that was stripped away by the last three centuries of science is being restored.

This movement is much more than a swing of the pendulum. The discoveries we are now making in energy science will permanently change the way we will view human life and the models we will use to describe it.

Meridian tapping is at the heart of this new movement. We are learning – or perhaps it is more accurate to say *relearning* – that the *energy system* of the human mind/body is a powerful engine that drives the way we think, feel, remember and experience. And it is extremely responsive to beneficial modification if we employ the correct intervention.

The beauty of the tapping method is that it places the means of intervention into the hands of everyday people. We all have access to it. Tapping is a gentle, non-invasive, yet extremely profound, way to directly and creatively reshape the very energies that enliven our minds, bodies and emotions.

As suggested in the last chapter, the possible uses for meridian tapping are immense and have scarcely been tapped as yet. When we look forward to a world in which tapping is widely known, accepted and practiced, it is easy to envision powerful, positive transformations in almost all of our institutions and relationships.

Tapping can focus and amplify the ability of people everywhere to help each other and themselves in an unprecedented fashion.

Meridian Tapping and the Future of Medicine

One of the most obvious arenas where meridian tapping will transform the status quo is medicine.

I think we can all agree that health care is in crisis. We have created a cumbersome, expensive and often violent system that focuses primarily on attacking disease rather than the promotion of wellness. Experts on all sides of the political fence acknowledge that this must change or become unsustainable. We need new paradigms and protocols. We need to become *pro*active rather than *re*active, preventive rather than palliative. We all need to assume more responsibility for our own wellbeing and to learn better ways to activate the natural healing mechanisms of the human body.

Humanity's new approach to wellness must involve gentle, non-invasive and preventive measures that dramatically reduce the likelihood of many of our present diseases. Dawson Church,

Ph.D., author of *The Genie in Our Genes*, points out in this important book that the day is fast coming when "Spiritual and emotional remedies will be the first line of defense, not the last. Sufferers will seek [energy-based] solutions *not* when they have *exhausted* all conventional means, but instead *before* they submit to the drugs and surgery of allopathic medicine." (p. 256)

He envisions a humane medical system in which "the most benevolent and least invasive therapy is used first." (p.304) There would then be "an escalation of interventions, using the simplest ones as the first line of treatment, and employing more drastic means only if the previous treatment is not effective..."

Meridian tapping will surely be one of these first-line interventions. If patients have at their fingertips (literally!) a simple and effective technique such as tapping, we can expect that many illnesses will simply take care of themselves. Providing an initial tapping session to a patient could change the course of untold numbers of medical treatments and reduce both cost and suffering. It would *shift* the patient's self-defeating beliefs and fears, rather than suppress them with prescription drugs.

As I look to the future of meridian tapping in medicine I can envision...

- Paramedics administering tapping on the spot to prevent shock and to enable patients to handle the trauma of an accident or sudden illness as they are transported to the hospital.

- Emergency room nurses leading patients through rounds of tapping while they wait for diagnosis, treatment and possible admission, thus making the pain more manageable and shifting the patient's outlook to one of hopefulness and cooperation.

- Closed circuit televisions in doctors' and dentists' waiting rooms, showing patients how to tap in order to cope with the many anxiety-producing situations that can occur during the waiting time.

- Practitioners in all medical fields administering tapping as routinely as they now record the patient's current medical status.

Meridian Tapping and Crisis Intervention

It is also easy to imagine meridian tapping becoming part of the standard protocol for crisis intervention at the site of natural disasters, accidents and in war zones. What a tremendous opportunity it offers to ameliorate trauma right on the spot, rather than wait until physical and psychological problems develop months or years down the road!

When some of us who are clinically trained applied meridian tapping to victims of the 9/11 disaster in the U.S., it far outperformed any of the conventional treatments being used for post traumatic stress. We did not, however, have *official* sanction for using it at that time because medical authorities and rescue teams did not recognize it as a safe and researched tool, so our ability to apply it was limited. But this will not be the case in the future. Meridian tapping is rapidly being approved and adopted in more and more conventional treatment venues.

When Red Cross and Search and Rescue workers are trained in meridian tapping and can make it available at the site of a disaster it will greatly mitigate the toll the disaster takes on everyone involved. Tapping will be used for traumatized victims of *any* sort, and is already being used in shelters for abused women. Used as a regular part of rehabilitation programs, it will help to handle addictions on a deeper level.

Meridian Tapping 101

Another area that will open up to meridian tapping in ways we cannot yet imagine is education. It is already being used on an individual basis to alleviate exam anxiety, performance anxiety and mental/emotional blocks regarding certain school subjects. I myself have used tapping to increase computer skills in a professional web designer. The rapidity with which he overcame his emotional blocks to using a certain computer language when we applied tapping to this problem was astonishing.

I can envision classrooms of the future in which teachers routinely ask students to tap as a group to allay anxiety before exam booklets are handed out. (Schools that want to increase their standardized test scores, take notice.) Already we are getting reports of school counselors who are conducting meridian tapping group treatment for severe behavior problems in schools. School counselor Syandra Ingram, for example, reports that tapping has given the best results she has ever had with recalcitrant students in a low-income, crime ridden district of her city.

I can see children disadvantaged by reading disorders, ADD and other learning disabilities practicing meridian tapping consistently along with other remedial measures. The introduction of tapping to college students under pressure will afford a major tool for educators and counselors.

Meridian Tapping in the Family and Community

I expect the everyday use of tapping to be widespread in the near future. One of the most striking features of this method is its ready availability to the average person. It requires no theoretical knowledge, special skills, or intellectual understanding. People from all walks of life and all levels of education can learn and benefit from meridian tapping.

It's exciting to imagine a time when parents and children will use tapping whenever a child experiences a nightmare, becomes angry at their siblings or gets into a homework struggle. Isn't this far preferable to allowing the distress of everyday incidents to fester within the child and family? Someday soon, parents may routinely and quietly tap on the child's comfort spots as they ask her to recount the problems of her day. Some parents are already doing this and it is proving remarkably effective. It nips the problem in the bud by eliminating emotional upset at its source.

I also predict that animal owners will soon learn to use tapping as a first measure to help pets in distress. This will not only create happier pets but more responsible pet owners and better neighborhood relations, as annoying habits like incessant barking, scratching or digging can often be completely arrested by using tapping.

An extraordinary aspect of this method is the way people of all ages instinctively share tapping with others in distress.

Gaining satisfaction through helping others is, it seems, an innate characteristic of human life. Surveys conducted on my website – in its special Explorers Center – show that a large percentage of people apply meridian tapping almost as often to others' problems as they do to their own. It is extremely gratifying to be able to bring help to others so easily and rapidly. What a lovely way to build community and create bonds of caring and friendship.

Meridian Tapping and the Human Spirit

The potential of using meridian tapping for spiritual purposes, for the deepening of human values and the fostering of a cooperative and peaceful world, is enormous. I can envision its widespread use amongst religious and humanitarian groups. We have seen how effective tapping can be at erasing hatred in a single individual. Imagine using it on a widespread scale to increase tolerance, compassion and nonviolent thinking.

Spiritual development is often blocked or greatly slowed down by persistent negative attitudes, thoughts and emotions. meridian tapping can be a tool for clearing the inner obstacles to achieving deeply satisfying spiritual growth in one's life.

The effectiveness of surrogate tapping has been demonstrated in innumerable individual cases (see the reports on Gary Craig's website, www.EmoFree.com). Is it so "out there" to imagine large groups of people doing surrogate tapping sessions to help their leaders come up with better solutions in peace negotiations and national policy meetings?

Might there even be a day when we all tap for the entire human race to help it evolve in a more loving, compassionate and peaceful direction?

The possibilities are breathtaking

Meridian tapping is a gift that we can give to ourselves and others that has almost no negatives involved. It is a gentle balm that has been made available to the human race at this time in history. I am proud to be part of the hope that it offers every one of us.

Special Resources

Areas covered:

- Meridian Tapping Internet Resources
- How to Locate Meridian Tapping Practitioners

Meridian Tapping Internet Resources

TheTappingSolution.com

This is where you can order your copy of *The Tapping Solution*, the feature film. You can get the latest information about the movie including information about participants and experts. Go now to receive a free ebook with articles from many of the experts featured in the film. Go to **www. TheTappingSolution.com**.

TappingInsidersClub.com

This is a sister site to TheTappingSolution.com. You can hear Jessica Ortner interview practitioners from all over the world. There are over 50 audios available on a huge variety of topics.

Go to **www.TappingInsidersClub.com**

TappingInternational.com

This is an online database located on a website that lists meridian tapping practitioners and workshops, and presents selected meridian tapping products. You'll be able to easily search for what you're looking for through a variety of different search criteria. One of the exciting functions of this site is the user ratings and feedback system which gives you information from other people regarding their experience with that particular practitioner, workshop or product so you can best make the right decision for your needs! Go to **www. TappingInternational.com**.

TappingCentral.com

This website is hosted by EFT Master, Dr. Patricia Carrington. It offers such major features as the Explorers Center where, using online surveys, your personal experience with meridian tapping can be shared with others and used to amass data that makes the practice of meridian tapping even more effective. This site contains huge amounts of information on meridian tapping, previews of Dr. Carrington's unique meridian tapping training materials, and many special offers, It is a major site for those who wish to think seriously about meridian tapping, why it works, how it can be improved upon, what is new and exciting in the field. Go to **www. TappingCentral.com**.

PatClass.com

This website contains a groundbreaking series of teleseminars by Dr. Patricia Carrington, Frontiers of Meridian Tapping. In these she introduces state-of-the-art methods of applying meridian tapping to personal growth, spiritual concerns, and many other innovations in the technique. Go to **www.PatClass.com**.

Emofree.com

This classic website is hosted by the founder of the meridian tapping technique EFT, Gary Craig. It is a major EFT resource containing literally thousands of reports by users worldwide on various uses of EFT. It also sells Gary Craig's masterful collection of original EFT training materials and gives access to his EFT Certification materials. Use its Search feature to find our just about anything you need to know about EFT's use and applications. Go to **www.emofree.com**.

AttractingAbundance.com

This website, hosted by EFT Master Carol Look, gives you up-to-date articles on the use of meridian tapping for abundance, addictions, pain control and other important specialty areas. It provides current information on Carol's teleclasses and workshops and a chance to explore her many outstanding products. Go to www.AttractingAbundance.com.

TappyBear.com

This appealing website introduces meridian tapping to children and their parents through the character of TappyBear, a loveable wise "friend" with whom children readily identify. Children learn the advantages of tapping by means of songs, coloring books, and other fun ways. A very effective site when you are considering introducing meridian tapping to children. Go to www.TappyBear.com.

Websites of practitioners who appear in the film *The Tapping Solution*

Helena Johnson. Meridian tapping practitioner in the film. **www.LivDelicious.com**

Carol Look. Meridian tapping practitioner in the film. **www.AttractingAbundance.com**

Steve Munn. Meridian tapping practitioner in the film and Owner/Director of the Retreat Center, Clear Point, featured in the film, a source of ongoing holistic workshops. **www.YourClearPoint.com**

Rick Wilkes. Meridian tapping practitioner who teaches EFT to the group in the film. **www.ThrivingNow.com**

Websites of Expert Commentators Who Appear in the Film

Jack Canfield – www.JackCanfield.com
Patricia Carrington – www.TappingCentral.com
Dawson Church – www.DawsonChurch.com
Donna Eden – www.InnerSource.net
Fred Gallo – www.EnergyPsychology.com
Bruce Lipton – www.BruceLipton.com
Carol Look – www.AttractingAbundance.com
Joseph Mercola – www.Mercola.com
Bob Proctor – www.BobProctor.com
Cheryl Richardson – www.CherylRichardson.com
David Rourke – www.DavidRourke.com
Norman Shealy – www.NormShealy.com
Carol Tuttle – www.CarolTuttle.com
Rick Wilkes – www.ThrivingNow.com
Joe Vitale – www.MrFire.com
Brad Yates – www.BradYates.net

Major Meridian Tapping Newsletters

Meridian Tapping Times.   This essential newsletter supplies a brief, lively, twice monthly report about what is going on in the world of meridian tapping and the latest innovations that you can use to enrich your meridian tapping practice. Edited by EFT Master Dr. Patricia Carrington, it is widely recognized as a source of in-depth information about meridian tapping. When you subscribe, you receive a bonus e-book by Dr. Carrington. Go to **www. TappingCentral.com**

EFT Insights. This classic newsletter edited by Gary Craig, Founder of EFT, is a "must" for all serious students of EFT. Published twice weekly, it is filled with fascinating reports and new hints by EFT users. To subscribe go to **www. Emofree.com**

Attracting Abundance with EFT. Dr. Carol Look's popular newsletter devoted to information about using meridian tapping to increase abundance and prosperity in your life. Go to **www.AttractingAbundance.com**

Tappy Times.   An entertaining and highly instructive newsletter that keeps parents and children up to date with the adventures of TappyBear and motivates children to use meridian tapping for many different children's issues. Go to **www.TappyBear.com**

How to Locate a Meridian Tapping Therapist

Because of the lack of centralization in meridian tapping training, it is important for anyone seeking help from a meridian tapping practitioner to do so with as much information on hand as they can obtain. Dr. Carrington's authoritative free e-Book entitled A Guide to Finding a Meridian Tapping Practitioner can be downloaded from her website www.TappingCentral.com. If you are searching for a suitable meridian tapping practitioner, we strongly recommend that you first print out and read this Guide. It will help you evaluate the names you can obtain from the major online lists of meridian tapping practitioners: the list of practitioners with performance reviews of their treatment approach (at www.TappingInternational.com); the list of Certificate holders from the EFT Certificate Program (www. TappingCentral.com) and Gary Craig's list of practitioners on his website (www.Emofree.com). Participation in any of these lists is voluntary, and the major lists partially overlap each other, but using them in conjunction with Dr. Carrington's guide you can readily locate qualified practitioners in your vicinity for in-office treatment, or worldwide for telephone therapy.

References

Achterberg, J. & Lawlis, G.F. (1980). Bridges of the Bodymind: Behavioral Approaches for Health Care. Champaign, IL: Institute for Personality and Ability Testing.

Ader, R., Felten, D.L., Choen, N. (Eds). (2000). *Psychoneuroimmu-nology – Third Edition*. New York, NY: Academic Press.

Baker, A. H. & Siegel, L. (2005). Can a 45 minute session of EFT lead to a reduction of intense fear of rats, spiders and water bugs? – a replication and extension of the Wells et al. (2003) laboratory study. Paper presented at the annual meeting of the Association for Comprehensive Energy Psychology, Las Vegas, Nevada.

Baker, A. H. (2008). An updated analysis of the results of the Baker-Siegek study. Personal communication to the author.

Benson, H. (1982). Body changes during the practice of g Tum-mo yoga (Matters Arising). *Nature*, 298: 402.

Byrd, R. C. (1988). Positive therapeutic effects of intercessory prayer in a coronary care population. *Southern Medical Journal*, 81 (7) 826-829.

Byrne, R. (2006). *The Secret*. New York, NY: Atria Books.

Carrington, P. (2000). *EFT Choices Manual*. Kendall Park, NJ : Pace Educational Systems.

Carrington, P. (2004). *EFT in Action for a Snake Phobia* (DVD).

Kendall Park, NJ : Pace Educational Systems.

Carrington, P. (2007). *Multiply the Power of EFT: 52 New Ways to Use EFT That Most People Don't Know About.* Kendall Park, NJ: Pace Educational Systems.

Carrington, P. (2008). *A Guide to TappyBear: How to Use Tappy for Your Child and Yourself.* Kendall Park, NJ: Pace Educational Systems, Inc.

Church, D. (2007). *The Genie in Your Genes.* Santa Rosa, CA: Elite Books.

Craig, G. (1999). *Emotional Freedom Techniques: The Manual (3rd edition).* El Paso, CA: Mediacopy.

Jahn, R. G. (1987). *Margins of Reality.* New York: Harcourt Brace Jovanovich.

Lipton, B. (2005). *The Biology of Belief.* Santa Rosa, CA: Elite Books.

Look, C. (2006). *Improve Your Eyesight with EFT.* Bloomington, IN: Authorhouse.

Look, C., Radomski, S., & Carrington, P. (2006). *The Key to Successful Weight Loss* (e-book within computer program *The Key to Successful Weight Loss*). Kendall Park, NJ : Pace Educational Systems.

McDonald, J. (2007). *Tapping Into Clarity: My Personal Journey Throughout the Filming of "The Tapping Solution"* (e-book). mcgolf@satx.rr.com.

Rowe, J. (2005). The effect of EFT on long-term psychological symptoms. *Counseling & Clinical Psychology Journal,* 2 (3), 104-111.

Swingle, P. G. & Swingle, M. K. (May, 2000). Effects of the Emotional Freedom Techniques (EFT) method on seizure frequency in children diagnosed with epilepsy (to contact Dr. Swingle go to www.SwingleAndAssociates.com).

Swingle, P. G., Pulos, L., & Swingle, M.K. (2004). Neurophysiological indicators of EFT treatment of post-traumatic stress. *Subtle Energies and Energy Medicine*, 151, 1, 75-86.

Wells, S., Polglase, K., Andrews, H.B., Carrington, P., and Baker, A. H. (2003). Evaluation of a meridian-based intervention emotional freedom techniques (EFT) for reducing specific phobias of small animals. *Journal of Clinical Psychology*, 59 (9), 943-966.